The Couples' Kama Sutra

THE COUPLES'
kama sutra

THE GUIDE *to* DEEPENING YOUR INTIMACY *with* INCREDIBLE SEX

Elizabeth McGrath

Illustrations by Gianluca Folì

SONOMA
PRESS

"You do not have to be good.
You do not have to walk on your knees
For a hundred miles through the desert, repenting.
You only have to let the soft animal of your body
love what it loves."
–Mary Oliver

To each of the brave individuals who have reached out to me through the ether and to those searching even now, looking to learn about themselves, discover more pleasure, practice self-love and healing, choosing valiantly, quietly, and courageously to let their bodies love what they love, you are my purpose. This is for you.

And to those in my life who love me and let me be "Me" with a capital *M*, shame-free. There are no words big or beautiful enough to describe my gratitude.

Contents

Introduction

SEX IS A FASCINATING ASPECT OF HUMANITY.

I believe that, and if you're reading this book, then you probably know it, too. So before I tell you about the incredible sex that will deepen the intimacy in your relationship, let's talk about how I came to find sex so fascinating.

In the sex education classes I attended in junior high through college, I was always interested in what kinds of questions my fellow students would ask, in how sex and sexuality were discussed or avoided. As a teenager, enthusiastic about disseminating accurate and open sex information, I began working at a phone hotline that served to educate, answer questions, and offer assistance on sex, body, and gender issues.

Not long after, I started a job at a shop called Good Vibrations, a female-friendly, education-based retailer that sold high-quality sex-positive products. Their mission was to provide nonjudgemental, accurate, and trusted sex information while enhancing people's sex lives and promoting healthy attitudes about sex overall. Working at Good Vibrations gave me a deep wealth of knowledge about sex and introduced me to the concept of shame-free sexuality.

Then I became a counselor at St. James Infirmary. I began to teach workshops, attend conferences, and travel around the world speaking about sex and sexuality in all its forms. When I saw firsthand that sex could be not only fun but also empowering, I wanted to share that transformative message with others wherever and however I could. I dreamed of making this my actual career, so I attended graduate school and received training in a variety of therapeutic methods, including emotion-focused therapy, cognitive behavioral therapy, and the psychodynamic approach, which helped form the basis of my own unique approach to the subject.

Throughout this period, I continued to teach, write, and educate people about sex, but I felt as though my passions for sex and sexuality existed alongside my social work rather than as its focus. It was only when I directed my attention toward my lifelong passion for dance that everything clicked. Being a dancer taught me about my body, which led me to learn and then start teaching yoga.

This, in turn, showed me what kind of work I was truly meant to do. Starting my somatic education solidified those instincts, and I suddenly understood how everything I was doing professionally and personally already intertwined and could work together to create a practice in Somatic Sexuality. After years of training with Somatica and the study of Hakomi Method and Experiential Therapy, I finally felt ready to take my unique style of sex therapy practice into graduate-level teaching and private practice with clients.

Those clients, to whom I am deeply grateful, have given me my greatest education and grown my work beyond anything I ever imagined. Each day my clients give me the gift of doing what I love most: helping people practice self-love and develop healthy and happy relationships that are fulfilling and sustainable, coaching people in removing barriers to the sex and relationships they want; and contributing to making the world more sex-positive and shame-free.

So here you are, accompanying me on that journey! I am here to support you in discovering your authentic sexual self, both on your own and while connecting with your partner. That is what this book is all about: introducing you to sexual experimentation, showing you how to create a lasting transformation, and helping you lay the foundation for incredible, true-to-you sex that deepens and fulfills your relationship. I'm a big fan of the saying *Doing things differently gets you different results,* and in reading this book, you will discover many opportunities to try new and different things and to learn from each experience. I hope you're as excited as I am.

Everyone Needs a Little Sex Therapy

As you may have gathered by now, I'm big on helping people have the great sex and relationships they want and deserve. That's why I have worked with hundreds of people to discover their wants and needs and communicate their feelings to those they love. My work is part traditional therapy, part sex education, part relationship coaching, and many parts somatic, all interwoven to meet the individual needs of each client—in this case, you.

When I say "somatic," I mean "of or relating to your body"—what you feel, sense, and experience. I like to say it's "everything from below the brain on down." Somatic work is a set of inquiry, practices, and perspectives that emphasize your physical awareness and your internal perceptions and experiences. Your body is where you gather physical and sensory information that tells you what we want and need to feel good, safe, and alive.

Most people spend a lot of time stuck in their heads, paying attention to their bodies only when they need immediate attention, like when they are hungry, ill, or in pain. One of the hallmarks of modern society is the ability to forget your body altogether: to be safe, comfortable, and happy without concern for physical discomfort. But when you do this, you disconnect from the potential for sensation and pleasure that you possess as a sexual creature.

My clients will often describe the best sex they've ever had along the lines of, "It just felt so good. I wasn't overthinking it, we were just connected. It was so passionate." This is what people mean when they talk about "incredible" sex. The big difference between their best sexual experiences and ones that felt more frustrating is how much time they spent in their mind versus their body.

That wrestling between mind and body is what brings clients to me. They want more connection, presence, pleasure, arousal, understanding. They feel as if they've struggled and suffered. They need a way to shift their experience. This book offers you a way to connect with the extraordinary body you have so you can begin to recognize it as the location of all that is good and delicious about being human and alive.

How to Use This Book

This book is structured like the sessions I offer to my clients. You'll learn the basics of embodiment, desire, and connection, and then you'll look at your relationship—the sex you are having and the sex you want to have. From there I invite you to push yourself a bit and integrate everything you have learned by trying great sex positions based on the *Kama Sutra*.

If you read this book carefully, you can expect to find a lot of new information about yourself and your partner. You'll learn more about what you want and need, how to connect more deeply, and how to feel fulfilled. You'll become more turned on and more in touch with your body.

Start by reading the book on your own. Notice what excites you. Then go through it with your partner and let them communicate what they like. You can play with the different combinations of talking, touching, and experimenting with sex positions, and you can come back to this book as a refresher to keep the fires burning, and as a therapeutic tool to keep you in touch with your body and connected to your partner. Explore how your body is feeling; the various sections may feel different for you on different days. All the sex positions I describe in this book can be combined with the advice about talking, touching, toys, and more—the combinations are endless.

Truly Incredible Sex

CHAPTER 1

The Spark

IT'S LIKELY THAT YOU MADE YOUR WAY TO THIS BOOK BECAUSE YOU WERE LOOKING FOR SEX POSITIONS and practices to explore, and the first thing that came to your mind was the *Kama Sutra*. I think it's awesome that an ancient Indian text—the oldest textbook of erotic love, dating back more than 2,000 years—is still highly relevant to modern life. The *Kama Sutra* has allowed so many people to connect to their sexuality beyond what might usually be seen as salacious or merely titillating. Its exposure in the West began in the sexually revolutionary times of the 1960s and 1970s, and it continued more deeply in the 1980s and1990s as the country experienced radical perception shifts around sexuality and relationships. It has become synonymous with experimenting with sex positions, from the basic to the downright acrobatic.

The *sutra*, or "narrative," was written by Vātsyāyana, but the *Kama Sutra* was distilled from the writing of several authors who came before him. The *Kama Sutra* was meant to educate its readers about many aspects of Indian cultural life during that time and was both an abstract and prescriptive thesis on finding a partner, power in marriage, adultery, drug use, the spiritual possibilities of different kinds of relationships, seduction, sexual and relational role reversal, intellectual and spiritual well-being, self-care, and grooming—in short, all things having to do with *Kama*, or love, desire, and pleasure, one of the main goals of Hindu life.

One of the most groundbreaking things about the *Kama Sutra* was its suggestion that sex is intended for pleasure and that this pleasure is one of the most direct paths to *Kama* itself. The *Kama Sutra* also argued that sex is a matter of culture, not just nature—an idea that is still considered relatively progressive today.

For Couples

Why should the foundations of the *Kama Sutra* be a jumping-off point for a very contemporary book about how to deepen your sexual intimacy?

I believe that people are often searching when it comes to sex and their sexuality—searching for how to have more, feel more, and keep the flame of their sexual self alive for as long as they choose. Although it's thousands of years old, the *Kama Sutra* focuses on many of those questions. It offers a timeless structure for experimenting with sex.

Over time, the initial sexual spark in your relationships can wane, and you might find yourselves looking back at the early days of your relationship, that "getting to know each other" stage when the sex was the most fun or closest to what you love. Or you might find yourselves in a place where you want something different out of life.

The author David Deida writes about the idea of "polarity" in relationships, and I often use that concept with clients to talk about what gives them a sexual spark. Sexual attraction is often a result of the differences that exist between you and your partner. It arises from the unknown, from new power dynamics and new risks. It stems from the tension of seeing a person who is separate from you and therefore exciting, and from the newness of simply getting to know someone. Later you create emotional attraction by bonding, building rapport, and discovering your common passions.

Dynamic relationships need both kinds of attraction to thrive, but it's common to swing in the direction of emotional attraction as you strive to be close to one another. You focus on trust and connection as you build your lives together. But you also need to maintain tensions and differences to feel excited and see that your partner can still thrill you.

A client once told me about seeing her partner across a crowded room: "It was almost like he was a stranger, and for a moment he wasn't my partner—he was so strong and confident." That's an example of this shifting polarity—a recognition of difference, a flash of separation that intrigues you and turns you on.

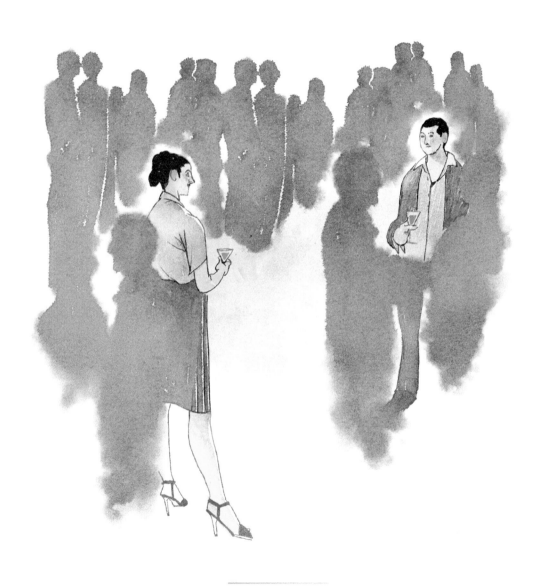

"It was almost like he was a stranger, and for a moment he wasn't my partner—he was so strong and confident."

To cultivate both emotional and sexual attraction, you must be willing to examine the way you observe and perceive each other. You must begin to embrace something new—even if that means confronting possible awkwardness and discomfort.

Why We Fuck

Sex is a stress reliever; sexual arousal releases a chemical in your brain that revs up your brain's pleasure and reward system and boosts your self-esteem and happiness. Studies have shown that sex can decrease blood pressure and keep your immune system healthy. Sex can also encourage your libido. If you've ever heard anyone say, "When I have sex, I seem to want it more," that is because having sex triggers the body's sexual responses, blood flow, and release of fluids and hormones—it signals a desire for more. Sex can help you with pain and pain management, and it may also help you sleep, by releasing the hormone prolactin during sex and after orgasm. Even touching and hugging can help your nervous system relax and cause your body to release feel-good chemicals. Having sex reminds you that you are sexy, sexual creatures. It helps you feel desired and appreciated and recognize one another as sexual beings. Sex creates connection, openness to exploration, and a desire for pleasure.

You have amazing bodies that are designed for pleasure. Everyone is capable of feeling good and achieving release in a variety of incredible ways. What more do you need? Sex!

GETTING "ENOUGH" SEX

One of the questions I get asked most is, "How often should we be having sex?"

First of all, I hate the word *should*. It suggests there is a rule that everyone needs to follow. Second, there is no meaningful average. Every couple is different and changeable from day to day. If you need to think in terms of numbers, a recent study done at the University of Toronto Mississauga showed that happiness in a relationship began to decline when couples started to have sex less than once weekly. For couples who had sex more than once weekly, happiness was not shown to increase in any measurable way, but below that frequency, connection, communication, and one or both partners' sense of well-being declined.

In my work I see couples not only in a variety of relationships but also in various stages of their time together. If there is one thing I can say with confidence, it is that sex and the need for it are aspects of life and experience that differ for every person. What I have found matters most is that a person or couple communicates about their needs for sex. It is completely common for one or the other of you to want more or less—rarely do people have the exact same level of sexual desire. Needs can also fluctuate over time, and they can be impacted by life, relationship issues, and physical and emotional factors. That being said, I have found that if the sex you are having feels connective and brings you emotionally closer to one another, having a little sex can lead to more sex.

I fall squarely on the side of *go for it*. Many people tend to get caught up in the idea of perfection, believing that sex has to happen a certain way for it to be great. But sometimes sex starts out awkward and ends up with the two of you panting, saying, "Why don't we do this more often?"

So to hell with the average. Talk with your partner about your desires and needs, find a balance, and explore a frequency that works for you both.

YOUR BODY IS NEVER WRONG

It is so common for my clients to feel fear and anxiety as they explore new ideas. I tell my clients there is no such thing as perfect sex or perfect communication. There is no doing it "right." Just be as true to you and as connected to your body as you can be.

Everything you do and try teaches you about your sexuality, what you and your partner want and enjoy. At which point do you feel excited, hopeful, connected, aroused, or warm in your body? Connect to that and allow yourself to move forward at a pace that feels possible. This is a great place to practice being gentle with yourself. Notice how you're judging your interests or wants—and never worry about saying or doing the "right" thing. You've got this! Take one step at a time and breathe into that awesome body; it's got all the information you need.

CHAPTER 2

Lighting a Fire

WHEN YOU THINK ABOUT SEX, CHANCES ARE YOU USUALLY THINK ABOUT ALL THE FUN STUFF AT THE END. But sex is about more than what happens when your bodies meet. It includes your turn-on and arousal, communication, flirtation, and the experience of secure attachment. This is your moment to learn how to experience all the ways your body feels pleasure and to explore some of the tools you already have for feeling it more intensely.

Embodiment

I believe embodiment is a deeply important aspect of sexual enjoyment. I believe it's the key to making your life truly incredible.

Embodiment may sound like a meaningless buzzword. You live in your body, so aren't you embodied already? Well, yes and no.

To be embodied is to be incarnate, to be corporeal, to fully inhabit that awesome body of yours. Although you live in your body, you don't spend much time *in* it—recognizing your sensations, being physically in the present moment. You usually stay in your mind, thinking, imagining, worrying, processing. But in addition to all the amazing and necessary things your mind does, it can also get in the way and keep you from fully inhabiting that incredible body of yours.

So how do you become more embodied? Here are some of the best ways to go deep and get the most out of your experience within yourself.

Breathing

Humans breathe more than 20,000 times a day, in and out without much awareness, which is why it's easy to take this function for granted. But actually, breath is one of the strongest natural connections between the mind and the body. If you can slow down, speed up, or shift your breathing, then you can slow down, speed up, or shift the way you experience pleasure. Breath work is at the center of all I do with my clients, and it's the most beneficial tool I have found for teaching people to feel more in every aspect of their lives—especially sex.

SLOWING DOWN

It is very common to feel nervous or anxious during sex. When you feel anxious, take a second to check in with yourself. If you want to have sex but you also want to settle your nerves, slowing down your breath is a great way to release some of that buzzy energy.

1. Notice what your breath is doing. When you're anxious, you tend to take quick, short breaths, which get stuck in your throat or upper chest area. Think of it like driving. If you're driving a car back and forth really fast on a tiny track, then it's not really going anywhere.

2. Count to eight, breathing in. Then count to eight, breathing out. Drive that car all the way into your body. Let your breath go all the way through you.

3. Notice how your shoulders come down and your throat relaxes. Don't worry if it takes many breaths before you feel this. Give yourself time to slow down. With slower energy comes more confidence.

4. When you start to worry, go back and focus on your breath. Feel it all the way through your body, long and slow. Go the distance.

FIRING UP

Where do you find the energy to be sexy? Again, your breath is a great way to get there.

1. Take note of what your breath is already doing at this moment. Maybe it feels slow and sluggish. Notice where you feel your breath flowing in your body.

2. Think of your breath as a fan for a flame in the center of your body. Every breath you take in fuels that fire and makes it grow—right in your belly, in your pelvis, in your cock or pussy or your perfect parts.

3. Relax your jaw and give your breath some sound. Let the sound of your inhaling resemble a gust of air coming in, and let the sound of your exhaling seem like a roar. If you find it hard to relax your jaw, shake your head and hair around, letting your face relax and your jaw hang as you shake.

4. Take your big breaths a bit faster, feeling the fire in your center expand and begin to heat you up right out of your fingers and toes, as if your body is catching fire. This warm energy is sexual energy. Even if all you feel are flickers here and there, don't judge these—let them grow and know that you can engage with touching yourself and your partner, making eye contact, flirting, all from this warm fire at your center. It was there all along—you just fanned the flames.

DEEPENING YOUR PLEASURE

Often people will tell me they get distracted during sex, thinking about what to buy at the grocery store or what they need to prepare for work the next day. It can be frustrating when you want to deepen your connection with your partner but instead you get stuck in your head. However, if you follow your breath into a physical spot in your body, you can draw yourself out of your head and into all the delicious sensations of sex.

1. Right now, take a moment to notice what your butt is doing. Are you sitting or standing? Can you feel the muscles of your butt? While you were reading this, you were thinking about the words and the concepts, but as soon as you concentrated specifically on your butt, suddenly there it was! This is the case with your entire body. Many people think of this as "focus," but it's more like awareness. Remember that your body is always present and there for you, just waiting to connect with your mind.

2. Now that you've raised your awareness of a particular part of your body, try breathing into that spot. Notice how you feel a bit more sensation there? Try flexing your muscles and breathing into those muscles. Notice that the sensation is slightly different. You can always do this during sex. Think about bringing your awareness into your cock or clit or butt or legs and then sending your breath to those spots—this is how you cultivate greater sensation.

3. Now that you've used your breath to reach those spots in your own body, think about bringing your awareness to your hands while touching your partner. Now you can experience double the sensation: everything your hands can feel (softness, warmth, smoothness, wetness, pulsing energy) and everything your body feels inside (excitement, turn-on, muscle contraction, calm connection). You can choose to focus on either of those sensations. If you want to drop in even deeper, try closing your eyes and slowing your touch—notice all the different, fun sensations your body suddenly picks up when you slow down and let yourself feel even more.

4. When you are being touched, either concentrate on the place you are being touched (the texture, feel, and sensation of the touch) or your heartbeat and the warmth in your belly and muscles. The more you bring your breath to the place of touch or to another place inside your body, the more those sensations will grow.

Don't get stressed out if you have trouble focusing. Breathing may sound easy, but it's something people rarely actually practice. Spend five minutes sending your breath to your butt and following its journey in your head. You'll get better at this. Be patient with yourself.

You can even ask your partner to help. Saying something as simple as, "Hey babe, feel this," while you're touching can help you focus your awareness. It can be a lot of fun to watch your partner feel more of these physical sensations.

Eye Contact

Shakespeare said "The eyes are the window to the soul" for very good reason. Looking into someone's eyes can tell you volumes about their mood, how they are feeling, and what they want. Eye contact can be especially powerful for connection and seduction. You can use it to feel closer, to flirt, to show your desire, and to tease.

THE INTENTIONAL LOOK

Try "intentional" eye contact. I tell my clients to practice this exercise as homework when they first come together at the end of a long day or after time apart. Stand facing one another, hold hands, and look into each other's eyes. It may feel awkward for a moment, but go with it. Really notice the color of one another's eyes and let any emotions that bubble up play on your face. It's okay to laugh

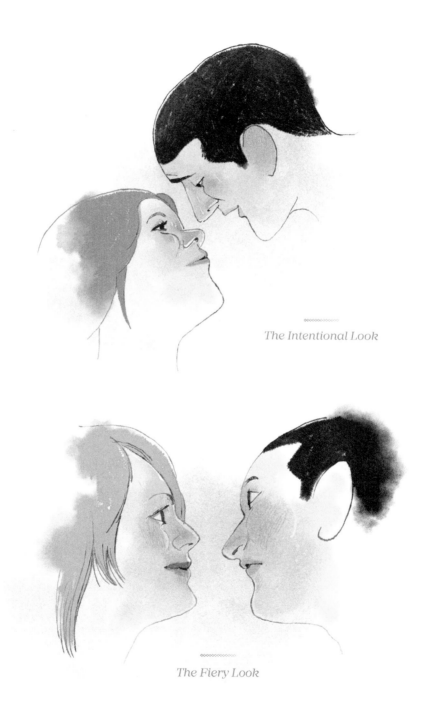

The Intentional Look

The Fiery Look

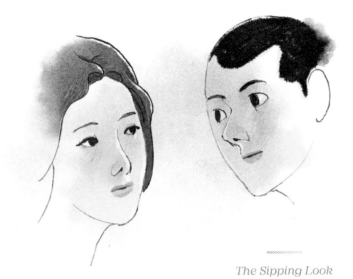

The Sipping Look

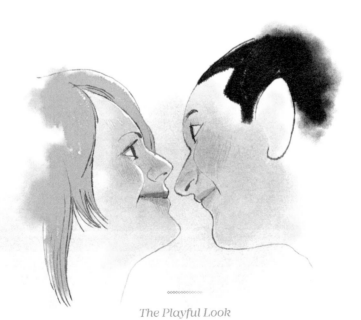

The Playful Look

and smile, but hold that connection for a full minute. You'll notice that even if it feels unusual to continue looking at each other, you will begin to feel "seen" and more connected. Make this a regular practice, and give it a try when you're arguing or wanting to diffuse tensions, too.

THE FIERY LOOK

Try "fiery" eye contact. First do the "Firing Up" exercise (page 20) to connect and boost your sexual energy. Then think about that desire coming through your eyes like a warm fire. As you make eye contact, think about what you want to do or have done to you. Channel your erotic thoughts and fantasies. You're sending your partner "I want you" vibes. If you feel your partner doesn't immediately sense your desire, don't be discouraged. Keep your energy strong to help them open up. Feel the depths of your fire and let it shine out of your eyes.

THE SIPPING LOOK

I encourage my clients to try "sipping" eye contact. It's like sipping from a delicious drink. You don't chug the whole thing all at once; rather, you just take small sips and enjoy. Make eye contact for a moment, let that flash of connection run through you, and then look away. Try watching your partner as they do everyday things like cleaning or cooking, and continue looking at them until they notice you watching. When they do, give a small smile and look away. Guaranteed, they will say, "What?" They'll be curious as to why you were looking at them. Dipping in and out of eye contact feels sexy and mysterious, as though you have exciting thoughts all your own.

THE PLAYFUL LOOK

Try "playful" eye contact. This is a lot like the Sipping Look but with a sweet and lighthearted twist. Imagine wrestling with your partner, grabbing their butt, and squeezing them—that electric energy can feel childlike and effervescent. Your eye contact will communicate, "I like you." Let yourself have fun with it. And if you partner doesn't immediately join you in that energy, keep going, feeling the desire within you, encouraging them with your looks to join in and have fun.

LOOKS TO AVOID

This may seem as if it goes without saying, but while you're playing with eye contact, you want to avoid rolling your eyes, closing your eyes and sighing, or getting angry and narrowing your eyes into a glare—unless you and your partner are consensually playing with angry energy. Remember how it feels to have someone look at you with these kinds of eye contact. If you get the sense that your feelings aren't being returned, gently pull back. Note your feelings and either communicate them openly in the moment or set them aside to express at a later time.

Talk

Communication is everything, but when it comes sexual needs and wants, it can sometimes seem like the biggest hurdle. You might feel shame or self-judgment about what you want, coupled with the pervasive belief that your partner is just supposed to "know" instinctively how to touch you, get you off, and bring you pleasure. Those assumptions can leave you feeling stuck and alone.

Often my clients will feel weird about communicating their needs and wants. They think, "This is so weird" or "This is such a big thing to want" or "My partner will think I am bossing them around" or "My partner will think they aren't doing a good job if I express this" or even "I'll never be able to have the experience I want, so why bother talking about it?" These responses are incredibly common. Why should you ask for what you want when even just thinking about it brings up so many conflicting feelings?

First of all, *your wants are important.* Read that again. Now say it aloud: *My wants are important.* Whatever you want—whether it's a particular way of being touched, a preferred sex position, something you fantasize about, or new feelings you're curious to explore—*your wants are important.*

In relationships, you teach people how to love you. When you connect with people, you begin to teach them how to bring you pleasure and joy. You're doing it without even realizing it. When you hold back during sex, your partner has to search for how to please you.

Communicating gives your partner the chance to touch you in that awesome way or to be a part of that sexy fantasy. When you talk with your partner about what you want, and then you receive it, this is what I call the "Closed Loop"—pleasure in every direction, flowing back and forth between you. This begins when you recognize that your wants are *important* and *necessary*.

Here is some language to get you started. Try practicing these lines in front of a mirror. Say them loudly and clearly, and then say them quietly from your belly, with your eyes closed. Check into your body and notice the thoughts that come up. There's no need to push the thoughts away, just let them rest there. Where do you feel it? What does it feel like? The fear and worry can wait—your desire is deep and important.

- "It really turns me on when you ..."

- "Yes. That right there, stay there just like that."

- "That's good and soft. Will you try doing it harder?"

- "I have this fantasy ... I'd like to tell you about it ..."

- "I've been thinking about some-thing lately and I'm wondering if I can share it with you ..."

- "The other night when we were fooling around, I noticed something I wanted ..."

- "I really like doing ... with you and I would like to do it ... (more/this way/at this time/longer)"

- "I used to enjoy ... and I'm wondering if we could try doing that together ..."

Talking about what you want doesn't always have to feel sexy. Sometimes it's important to say how you're feeling, even if you're worried or fearful:

- "I'm feeling nervous to talk about this with you ..."

- "I'm worried that if I express a want, it might cause you to feel less, and I don't want that ..."

- "It's challenging for me to say this because ..."

- "I'm trying to be more vocal about this. I wanted you to know, so we can get into it together."

If You Feel Pressured

Are you feeling like sex is a big event and it's hard to know if you can offer your complete self from start to finish?

Try looking at sex as a spectrum of possibilities and discuss it with your partner that way. Often people feel like they can't flirt with their partners if they aren't prepared to offer them the full monty. While this perspective is very common, it cuts out all the possibilities that can help you feel hot, intimate, and connected. Touching, flirting, quickies, snuggling, and foreplay can be fun and satisfying on their own.

I like to tell my clients that sex is a big box of donuts. There are many different kinds of donuts in the box. Most people think of sex as only two or three donuts—flirting, foreplay, intercourse—and they feel pressure to offer the whole box or none at all. But when you realize that all the donuts in the box are equally delicious, you start to consider which flavors you want to taste at different times; maybe these two flavors today and a different three tomorrow. And with each donut, you can eat the whole thing or just a take a few bites. When you are hungry, a single taste is better than none at all. You can feel good about all the flavors and bites you have to offer.

HOW TO TALK DIRTY

Dirty talk includes anything that seems off-limits, as well as words and phrases that fall outside of your comfort zone. The bad news is, most people are unpracticed at saying these things. The great news is, the taboo nature of the language is exactly what makes it hot, and the more you practice it, the easier it gets.

Let yourself embrace the dirtiness by repeating these phrases over and over to yourself, aloud. Then bravely say them to your partner in a moment when you're getting turned on:

- Try out words like *pussy, cock, dick, cunt, ass, clit, hole,* and *fuck*. A great starting formula is to add a racy word into a positive sex statement. Telling your partner when something feels good is an easy way to try out new words.

- When you feel comfortable with those words, add some action verbs: *use, take, own, bang, slam, break, stretch, have.* Use these to describe what you want or comment on what is happening in the moment.

- Once you pass the first few go-rounds with dirty nouns and verbs, you might want to try the next step of using dirty roleplaying words: *slut, whore, daddy, master, bad girl, bad boy, fuck toy, slave, bitch.*

If certain words immediately turn you off, you'll know instantly that those words are not hot for you. If this is the case, move on! You don't need to talk dirty to be able to have incredible sex. But if you find that spark of interest, let yourself follow it—some really hot sexcapades could be in store if you give it a try.

You might wonder how to tell if your partner is enjoying your dirty talk. Just like all types of sexual exploration, dirty language is all about connection and consent. Do you get the vibe that they like dirty words? Have they expressed interest or made comments that give you that feeling? Connect to what you know about them and what it feels like to be with them. Do they love romance and sexual softness? Then start with the easiest and most basic level of dirty talk. If they're into things a little more rough and rompy, try escalating your dirty talk and notice how that goes over. Your instincts about your partner matter, so go ahead and trust them while gently feeling it out.

For the roleplaying words, which can be degrading in other contexts, consent is critical: Get your partner's explicit approval before trying those. For example, "I want to call you dirty things. What do you think?"

Always avoid the following words: *stupid, ugly, fat, worthless,* and *dumb.*

When in doubt, go slowly. And as always, when you want to know what you partner likes, ask them! If they connect to your energy, you will feel it right away.

Foreplay

Sometimes, once you find what works and what your partner likes, you settle into a routine with one another. But foreplay can remind you of all the options you have. It can bring you back to your creative, sensual energy and make you feel new again. Remember that your bodies are always changing and capable of experiencing and enjoying new things. So try making your foreplay the main event, and really take your time with each kind of play.

Imagine you're touching your partner for the very first time. Even if you know them incredibly well, see what new sensations you can pick up about their skin, the feel of them, their smell, taste, and energy. Experiment with putting all these different play options in a new and different order. I like to call this energy the "Sex Lab." In this "lab," I encourage my clients to mix and match. I tell them just to have fun and see what happens when they get an idea for an experiment and play it out. If you find yourself getting concerned about doing it well or "right," just focus on your embodied breath exercise (see "Breathing," page 20); follow your breath back down into your body to feel all your amazing sensations.

EMBRACING

When you embrace, almost your entire body is touching another person. In foreplay, this full-body touch allows you to feel the energy of your partner's body. If you're standing in an embrace, think about feeling your feet on the floor, then extend your feeling to all the places where your body touches your partner. Really take them in, noticing how it feels to be so close.

If you're lying down in an embrace, see if you can enfold your partner or allow yourself to be enfolded by them. Try melting into each other. Notice everything that you enjoy about it. Let yourself move and shift in ways that feel good. Feel your breath all the way through your body, and breathe into your partner.

KISSING

I'm a huge fan of kissing. There is something so sensual and intimate about bringing our mouths together. Our breath is our life force and the energy that brings us into our body, so the joining of our breath with another person's is incredibly powerful.

Kissing is a fun opportunity to play with each other. Begin by slowing down and really noticing what you feel—lips, tongues, throats, chins, noses, everything soft and warm, maybe the tickle of a mustache or the sharpness of a gentle bite. When you slow down, you notice more. Try gently touching tongues, pressing your lips together, sucking on your partner's bottom lip, or pulling back a moment to feel your breath.

Take your time. Enjoy. If you feel your partner speeding ahead, bring a hand to the side of their face or the back of their neck, slow your breath, and gather them into your energy. Feel yourself getting more ravenous? Show your partner how badly you want them. Feel the power of your breath and theirs, and lose yourself to what feels good and what you love about it.

OUTERCOURSE

Otherwise known as "dry humping" (but come on, we can do better than that, right?), this is the super-hot activity of grinding, rubbing, and rolling around with one another. If you've ever done it before, you'll remember how quickly the energy gets charged up.

Try switching up positions. Take turns being on top and lying next to one another. See how you can find knees, thighs, and butts to grind on by scissoring your legs. Feel how much you want your clothes off, but keep them on and let that intensity build. Feeling a bit frustrated and ready to tear at each other? Good. On the other hand, if it feels slow and slightly awkward, see if you can hang out, explore what's there for you, and let yourself laugh while you give it a try.

UNDRESSING

Taking off your clothes can be an incredible tool for charging sexual tension. Even if you have seen someone naked countless times before, there is something so hot about imagining what they look like under their clothes and watching as those items of clothing come off one by one.

Try laying your partner down and slowly taking off their clothes one piece at a time, unwrapping them like a present. Or gradually undress for your partner, letting them watch. You can also stand and undress each other, looking at each exposed part and considering how that turns you on. Undressing is its own form of seduction.

MASSAGE

Massage is amazing. Studies have shown that touch can ease stress, speed up our healing, boost our mental health, and improve our sleep. Massage taps into several of the things I have talked about in this book: sensory awareness, embodied touch, experimentation with pace, energetic connection, and playfulness. When you take time to touch each other's bodies in an intentional way, you immediately feel closer.

Set aside some time to touch each other in exploratory ways. I like to tell my clients to plan a time to "arrive" together, when they can show up and be present with one another. If you want to try touching more firmly or use pressure, make sure you have a good lotion or body oil handy that allows your hands to glide smoothly over skin and rub more deeply into areas that are fun to touch.

You may think you already know how to touch your partner, but try to notice the warmth and texture of their skin, paying attention to how and where you want to touch. Use long strokes with your fingertips and the palms of your hands.

BATHING

One of the first homework assignments I give my clients is to spend some time in the bath or shower just noticing how the water feels on their skin, experiencing the warmth moving down the length of their bodies. I tell them

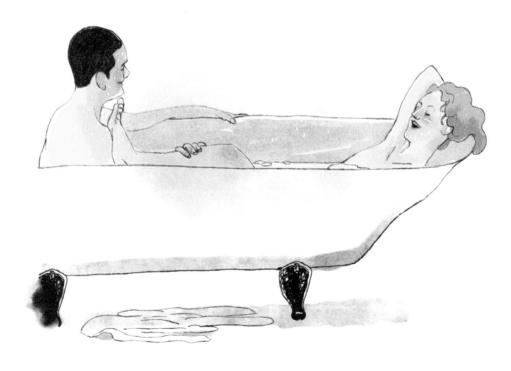

One of the first homework assignments I give my clients is to spend some time in the bath or shower just noticing how the water feels on their skin.

to connect to each place they feel the water, enjoying it and spending time with those sensations.

Now add another person to that experience. With a second person, there is suddenly twice as much to feel, sense, and enjoy. Notice the water on your skin and on your partner's skin. See how it feels to have their hands on your wet skin, and your hands on theirs. Touch each other's dripping hair and try slow, damp kisses. Soaping each other up and cleaning one another can add another dimension of super-sexy play. Take your time running soapy suds all over each other's bodies, and use your hands or a washcloth to clean one another.

Do you feel yourself getting turned on? Follow that feeling. If you start to want more intense oral sex or penetration, communicate with your partner about what feels good. Water can sometimes wash away the body's natural lubrication, so replenish that with lubricant, or take your play out of the water and onto dry land when you're ready to move on.

Know what else is great after a bath? Massage (see above)! Warm, damp skin can be great for rubbing and enjoying. Slowly towel each other off or have your partner sit and watch while you slowly dry off, moving the towel over every part of your body.

CHAPTER 3

Fuel for the Flames

SO YOU'VE BEEN FIGURING OUT WHAT YOU LIKE, WHAT FEELS GOOD FOR YOU AND YOUR PARTNER, and now you're ready to turn up the heat. Think of this chapter as adding extra spice to an already nourishing meal. Enjoy!

Spontaneity

One of the reasons sex feels so exciting early in a relationship is because we feel as if it could happen anytime, anywhere. Many clients ask me how to "get that back," and I say there is no "getting it back"—there is only "getting it forward." You can approach every moment with a sense that all kinds of sex are possible.

Spontaneity is about letting go of the notion that there is a perfect moment for sex. In a relationship, we can get fixated on doing sex "right." Comfort, safety, and support are all important, but focusing on them can make spontaneity feel impossible.

One great way to explore being spontaneous is to look at all the erotic possibilities that exist in day-to-day life with your partner. When can you reach out and sensually touch their body, grab them, squeeze them, push them up against a wall and make out? Whether or not you have intercourse, there are so many ways to show your desire. The best part about spontaneity is the feeling that sex can happen at any time. When you're overthinking the perfection of the moment, relax. Just show your partner that you've got sex on your mind. Remember other times you've been spontaneous about having sex. The repetition of that moment can bring back great, hot memories and guide you once again.

Try touching, grabbing, and sharing sensual talk in familiar places at unexpected moments, like while one of you is cooking, watching a show, or getting ready for bed. This way you can experiment with one element of spontaneity—breaking a routine—while staying in a place that feels safe.

Locations

Once you've broken your usual routine with spontaneous sex, take it out into the wild for another big surge of excitement. Pull your partner into the bathroom at a restaurant, take them into the trees for a hot make out session, or linger in the car and feel every inch of their gorgeous body. Your life is a playground of opportunities, offering a broad spectrum of sexy moments with your partner. Remember, it feels good to be desired.

Why would you want to take sex out of the bedroom and into the wild? Excitement! It's risky to have sex in public places. You might get caught. What would happen if you did? Most of the time the risk is purely theoretical, but the possibility makes it exciting. There is also something really hot about not being able to keep your hands off one another or wait until you get to a private place.

Where to try it? Elevators, restrooms, extra bedrooms at parties, parks, off-roading in nature areas, secluded alleys (busy alleys? I mean . . .), beaches, backyards, department store changing rooms . . . really just about anywhere can be a thrilling place for some hands-down-the-pants action, and an easy way to slip into intercourse.

But beware: Public areas are fundamentally nonconsensual—the people who might see you have not agreed to witness your fun. Public exposure may also be considered a crime, depending on where you live, so make sure you weigh in that risk. Also, public sex is sometimes less comfortable—it can mean less body lubrication and more physical contortions.

Personally, I'm a big fan of playing with sex somewhere semi-public: feeling each other up under the dinner table at a restaurant, fondling in the back row at the movies, flirting and grabbing in the back of a taxi. This can charge up your sexual energy, and as soon as you get somewhere private, you unleash it on each other.

Food

Food and sex are a great combination. They both nourish your body and stimulate your senses, satisfying your biological needs and emotional urges. Food can be incredibly seductive. Think about how good it feels when you're really enjoying your food: digging into it, moaning with pleasure, abandoning yourself to the taste, texture, and pure joy of consumption and fulfillment. We get the same energy from great sex.

Pay attention to the way you prepare food. Cooking is full of sumptuous opportunities for embodied awareness and touch. Close your eyes and really taste and smell what you're making. Try different parts of the dish before they go into the pan or oven. Feed your partner a bite or two.

It helps to engage the senses. Share foods that are hot, soft, cold, crunchy, and smooth. Use as many of your senses as you can employ. If you're feeding your partner or licking food off their body, start with simple flavors that are sweet or salty; avoid spicy or bitter foods unless you know your partner is really into them. Alternate back and forth between sweet and salty to feel the variation in taste.

Kitchens, dining rooms, and places where you can roll around and possibly get messy are great for first outings so you can go wild and don't have to worry about making a huge mess. Did you get messy? Grab each other and head to the shower or bath where you lick each other off. Use warm water and smooth soap to get everything squeaky clean.

When you play with food, you want to avoid anything going inside your body (other than the mouth) to prevent infection and complications. And remember, nothing without a flared base inside a bum! (Also, open bottles up the rear can have a suction effect, which can be dangerous.) When you're done with your food play, make sure that most of the sugary, salty, creamy, or sticky parts are all cleaned off so you can touch and penetrate wherever you like without concern.

Toys

Occasionally, clients express concern that their wanting to bring a toy into sex will make their partner feel intimidated or deficient in some way. I encourage people to communicate their thoughts about toys and props along the lines of pleasure. For instance, "This turns me on so much, I want to bring that extra pleasure to our play." Or, "I love when you . . . and using my vibrator there would take me over the edge." Remember that your wants and needs are important, and by communicating your desire to use a toy, you are creating an opportunity for an even deeper sensory experience for both you and your partner.

Shop together! If you want to use toys and props with your partner, picking them out together can really add to the heat of the experience. Shopping is a low-pressure opportunity to talk about trying new things. It also provides a chance to assuage any intimidation or worry about how the toy will feel or look. Jump on the computer and find a sex toy retailer that sells products you like, and ask your partner if anything catches their eye. Are they still a bit nervous? Suggest a trip to the store so you can touch the toys that interest you. Look at all the possibilities on the shelves. The sex toy world is your oyster!

If you feel a bit overwhelmed by all the options, try a kit. Massage kits, bondage kits, and vibrator kits all offer smaller and more introductory sizes of items you might be curious about or want to try. Introducing sexy new things in kit form can help you experiment before you commit, and this strategy can also let you spend less money before you buy the full-size version. Talk about experimenting with each of your new gadgets, seeing what you like, what is fun, what makes you laugh, and what turns you on.

What are the best items for your sex toolbox? I'll give you my top seven. If you feel intrigued or a little aroused as you're reading, that's a good sign you should give the item a try.

LUBE

Yup, this is considered a sex toy! And it's the most popular and frequently purchased of all sex toys. Know why? Because it's awesome.

Lube is the number one product I recommend to clients for regular use in their sex lives, both in their solo play and with partners. So much of what you enjoy sexually is about rubbing, grinding, and skin-to-body connection. Lube provides a smooth, slippery buffer for all that contact to feel easier, more comfortable, more sensitive, and more pleasurable. It's a great way to signal to your partner that you're prepping your body for more.

But you might say, "Elizabeth, shouldn't lube be unnecessary if I'm excited enough, and won't my partner think I'm not into them if I use it?" It's a great question and a common worry. I tell clients that even if you're feeling really turned on, lube can add to the sensation and allow you to go longer and feel more. You certainly don't have to do it—but try it. You'll want to!

Also, all bodies are different. Every person with pussy parts lubricates differently, and things like menstrual cycles, medication, stress, and how you're feeling can affect your lubrication from one day to the next. The unreasonable belief that wetness is a direct measure of turn-on is, thankfully, going the way of the erection-based turn-on, but nevertheless, it is still something we think about occasionally. (You can be super turned on and your body can respond in a myriad of ways, not all of them including wetness or an erection.) The cycle of arousal takes time, and your body may come around at its own pace. Go with that! And when you want to be wetter or you want the sex itself to be wetter, reach for the lube. Lube sometimes has the jump-start effect of creating more of your body's own wetness, which can feel great.

For anal sex, keep in mind that the anus does not self-lubricate the way a vagina might. Lubrication is a must for safety and pleasure.

You have a few different kinds of lube to choose from:

SILICONE Has unmatched slickness and staying power—it will not dry out. It is hypoallergenic, will stay on in water, washes off easily with soap, and will not be absorbed by your skin. These qualities make silicone lube great for long-lasting slipperiness, for body parts that don't make their own wetness (such as the anus and breasts), and for use in friction play and in water, like in the shower, pool, or hot tub.

WATER-BASED It's often thicker and has more of a cushiony feel than silicone, and it can be found in a variety of textures and thicknesses. Water-based lube can dry out much faster than silicone-based lube, as water-based lubes are absorbed by the skin. But unlike silicone, it can be instantly revived with a little water or saliva, and it rinses off easily without soap. It's safe to use with all toys, even silicone ones, and it's a great option for anal play because of its thickness.

FLAVORED Good for oral sex—it adds a fun flavor to mouth and hand play, though flavored lubes often contain sugars and glycerin, which can present problems if they get inside your body. A good rule of thumb is to let yourselves go wild with flavored lube if you're going to be removing all of it with your mouth. Start over with regular water-based or silicone lube for sex or if you'll be popping a condom over the sticky stuff.

OILS I get asked about natural oils all the time, and I encourage experimenting with them for massage and sensuous touch, but I do not recommend them for penetrative sex. Oil can damage latex, which means it's not safe for use with most condoms and dental dams. Also, different bodies react differently to oils internally, so it can be a bit hit-or-miss to figure out which ones will feel fine and sexy and slippery and which ones could present allergic reactions.

Ready to introduce lube into your sex life? A first-time user should start by keeping the bottle close at hand. When you and your partner are getting worked up, pour a small amount of lube (start with a dime-size amount, adding more as you go) into your palm. Rub it between your hands and fingers to warm it up. If you're using it on a cock or strap-on, slowly spread it over the tip and work your way all the way down the shaft. Use your slippery fingers on yourself or have your partner return the favor. When using a condom, you can increase the sensation by adding a drop into the tip of the condom before rolling it on, then smoothing some more over it before penetration.

VIBRATORS

Nowadays, there are about a million vibrators on the market, each one offering something different in the way of size, speed, power, shape, and where exactly it was designed to go. Let's start with the basic ones for outside use and work our way "in":

BULLET VIBES Small and handheld, either battery operated or rechargeable. Compact and with variable speeds, these can be fun to use during sex because you hold them against you, and you can cup them to one spot in most sex positions.

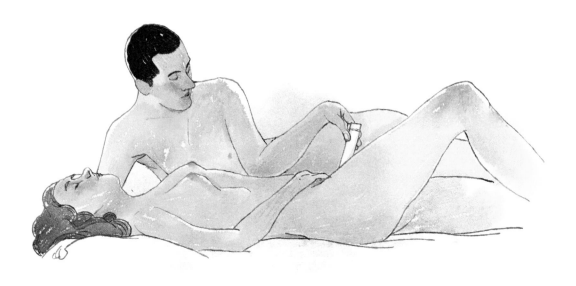

*Nowadays, there are about a million vibrators on the
market, each one offering something different*

VIBRATOR SHAPES Made of silicone or plastic and often shaped to be held along the body, these can be rechargeable or battery operated and may be larger and difficult to hold completely in the palm of the hand. The bigger ones will be stronger and more powerful, offering more speed options.

WAND VIBES These are the big boys that either plug into the wall or need to be connected to a rechargeable base. These vibes includes the mythical Magic Wand and are the ones you are most likely to hear about, because they are often quite powerful and get you off more quickly than smaller vibes. These can be too strong for some bodies, but if you love powerful vibration, there really is nothing better.

G-SPOT VIBES You'll know these by their curve. Often shaped like a gentle *C*, these are designed for insertion, and they work the G-spot while angling the smooth tip up and toward your belly button in whatever position you find yourself. They're often made of a firm material, like nonporous plastic or silicone. Look for ones with a removable vibe, so you can take that part out, if you like.

THE RABBIT Another type of vibe that has made its way to our cultural consciousness due to television shows and word of mouth, the Rabbit-style vibe is designed for internal use. The shaft spins, and so does a part designed to stimulate the clitoris. These vibes can feel great for some bodies and less great for others. They offer options that the standard vibe doesn't. If you're someone who loves penetration and sensation variety, you might want to give this one a "spin."

PARTNER VIBES Relatively new on the scene, these vibes are designed to provide stimulation for both partners. They look like a *U* and go inside the upper part of the vagina, with one part of the vibe stimulating labia and clitoris, and the other side providing stimulation to the penetrating partner. These can be a lot of fun but also hit-or-miss in terms of both partners feeling the stimulations.

DILDOS

Dildos offer you the option of penetrating or being penetrated by your partner in a variety of different ways. I encourage my clients to think about how fun it could be to use a dildo on their partner and see things they can't see when they're penetrating with other parts of the body. Dildos come in a myriad of sizes, shapes, and colors, so you can experiment with what feels good inside your body. Try sucking on your dildo as a tantalizing show for your partner. Use it on yourself while they watch or for extra penetration during sex.

My two favorite materials for dildos are glass and surgical steel. Both are nonporous, so they are easy to clean and you don't have to worry about bacteria collecting or the material degrading over time. Use only water-based lubes with silicone toys, and try gently warming them in warm water before each use. Glass and surgical steel toys warm even better inside the body. You can also warm them in water or by wrapping a warm cloth around them beforehand. Look for dildos that are visually appealing to you, and try different lengths, shapes, and sizes to discover what you like best.

COCK RINGS

For partners with cocks and those wearing strap-ons, a cock ring can add an extra level of sensation. Designed to go around the cock—either around the shaft or around the shaft and underneath the balls—cock rings can be used to maintain an erection, vibrate to provide stimulation, or both. Slip it on around the base of your shaft and bring it gently beneath your testicles while you are semi-erect. Partners can help with this as part of foreplay, and a little lube will help, too. Make sure the ring either snaps on or is super stretchy, or have a pair of safety scissors handy if it gets too snug and can't be easily pulled off.

If you use a vibrating cock ring, try it around the base of the shaft, aiming the vibrator to stimulate either the very sensitive underside of the cock or your partner during penetration. Most vibrating cock rings have battery-operated vibes, so check out how strong a vibration you like, and keep in mind that if you're using it to stimulate your partner's body, you'll want full body contact and a bit of grind.

SEX PILLOWS AND SHAPES

Sex shapes can be revolutionary. When you and your partner are able to angle your bodies in all the ways you want, things suddenly open up and sensory parts connect in ways you didn't even know were possible. You get to relax into the incredible moments you are experiencing, rather than having to hold your muscles in specific ways to get off. This book will introduce you to many positions that can be supported by various wedge shapes and pillows designed to move your body up, down, sideways, and upside down. The best sex shapes have water- and liquid-resistant coverings that can be removed and machine-washed.

BUTT PLUGS

Anal play is an equal-opportunity pleasure, and a great way to explore it for the first time is by using a butt plug. Awesome for folks of all genders, butt plugs come in many different shapes and sizes. They utilize a flared base to allow the toy to sit inside the anus, giving it a gentle stretch while not getting lost inside the body. Butt plugs are best in a nonporous material such as silicone (soft), glass (smooth), and surgical steel (very hard but warmed by the body). When in doubt, start small or purchase a kit that gives you options for different sizes. Some butt plugs can be used in addition to other kinds of penetration, but go slow and find out how much sensation feels good.

BONDAGE TAPE/RESTRAINTS

In sexual situations, bondage brings in a dynamic of power play that can be incredibly sexy (see Dominance/BDSM, page 44) and offers possibilities for roleplay, tension, and resistance. A great item for beginning with restraint play is bondage tape. It looks a lot like a roll of duct tape, except that it magically peels and then sticks back to itself without sticking to skin, hair, or sensitive parts of the body.

Thin and plastic, this tape is a fun way to restrain wrists, ankles, breasts, and cocks and to strap bodies to beds. Keep in mind that it is somewhat stretchy, so if you're interested in preventing your partner from getting free, this is a beginner-level restraint item. Also keep in mind that, though it has a bit of give, you are able to wrap it tightly, so leave a bit of room between the tape and the part of the body you are wrapping, and keep safety scissors on hand in case a tangle occurs or your partner needs to be freed quickly.

Other good restraint items include leather cuffs, bed-bondage straps, long leather belts that can wrap around the body, and soft rope that is machine washable. Clients ask me about handcuffs all the time, and while those can be fun for roleplay, they can be hard on wrists and tricky to remove quickly. If you love the idea of handcuffs, consider cuffs that are wider and cover more of the wrist and ankle area, as these options offer less risk of cutting off blood flow.

Dominance/BDSM

Remember when I spoke about sexual tension, and how a bit of risk and power shifting between you and your partner can fuel attraction and revive that thrill of newness (For Couples, page 14)? Playing with dominance and submission and incorporating S&M into sex can be a great way to add those tensions.

EXPLORE YOUR ROLES

There are so many ways to play with power dynamics. BDSM stands for bondage, discipline/domination, submission/sadism, and masochism. Under that broad and sexy umbrella are a ton of different ways to play with those elements. Spend some time considering a few of the roles you might want to assume:

- Dominant/submissive
- Master/slave
- Owner/pet
- Age play: Mommy/daddy/little angel/bad little boy/little girl

- Nurse/patient
- Teacher/student
- Sadist/masochist

When you first think about these, you'll get an immediate physical response of "mmmm yeah," "hmmmm no," or "uhhhh maybe." Follow that feeling—it contains good information about your needs and desires.

TRY IMPACT PLAY

Spanking is a classic, but there are so many ways to play with impact, pain, and discipline. Consider your hand, a flogger, a paddle, a riding crop or cane, as well as household items you may already have, such as a binder or clipboard, a towel for snapping, kitchen tools like a spatula or whisk, and the ever-awesome hairbrush. Start slowly, experimenting with sensation, as you feel your pleasure and your partner's responses.

ENJOY YOUR PARTNER

Often in relationships, we can get set in our ideas and perceptions of who our partners are and find it difficult to imagine them outside of these character- istics we feel we have come to know so well. One of the most alluring parts of BDSM and power play is experiencing our partners in new ways that feel foreign. Check in with your feelings from time to time, and let your partner try to move through any awkwardness while they explore their role and their feelings about it. Most of all, enjoy the newness of trying unfamiliar things with someone you're passionate about.

Endless Ways to Get Intimate

WELCOME TO YOUR NEW *KAMA SUTRA* PRACTICE! THINK OF THIS PART OF THE BOOK AS YOUR own personal sex gym; you've learned the basics, and now it's time to unleash yourself on all the equipment, try every single workout, and play around . . . crazy, sexy fun is at your fingertips!

On the following pages, you will find 41 positions designed to help you attain the energy, sensations, and pleasure you most desire. For each position, I've included an explanation on how it works, instructions on how to explore it, and a few specifics on what I think you will totally love about it. Check out the level of difficulty (1 is the easiest, 5 is the hardest), notice if the illustration intrigues you or turns you on, and then dog-ear that page to try it ASAP! Read through each of the positions with your partner or on your own. Make a little mark next to the ones you want to try, and have your partner do the same. Consider starting with the poses you both were equally excited about. Where you differ in your choices, take turns trying one person's picks, then the other's.

Remember all you have learned about communication, embodiment, breathing, and energy exchange, and keep in mind that you can always return to any part of this book for a refresher before experimenting with a new position.

Have fun! This is all about the spectrum of pleasure—from playful to intimate to powerful to racy to energetic, pleasure that feels a little bit good to really, *really* good. Let yourself enjoy anything that arouses your senses, and gently challenge your own boundaries as you discover more and more. I'm so excited for you to dig in and savor all that is here for you!

Pick Your Flavor

Wondering where to begin? The positions are grouped in the following chapters according to the type of energetic and physical exploration they might offer you. Notice the description at the beginning of each chapter, which defines the mood of the positions, and see if that's the energy you want to create. I encourage you to try all the different positions and to vary the type of sex you're having according to the message you want to send to your partner.

If you try a position and its energy feels different than how it was presented in the description, just go with it! Every relationship and body is unique, so sometimes a seemingly soft, intimate position will bring up a surprising amount of strong energy and hot power play. Don't fight it; celebrate that you've discovered what turns you on about the pose and what it does to your body.

Each of these chapters offers you a structure to play with, but make that play your own. Use these sections for inspiration, according to what you are feeling and what you want most. See aspects of a position you think you can improve? Off-road it! This book is fodder for your individual brand of pleasure. My greatest hope is that you will love this book, use it often, and eventually expand on these positions and concepts to create your own robust sexual repertoire.

Endless Ways

Who doesn't love a chart? Sometimes the sheer number of sexual options can feel so overwhelming, we don't know where to begin or what we really want.

At the beginning of each chapter, I will give you a chart that includes verbal and physical actions that will enhance your experience with the sex positions. These charts distill a lot of the basic foundations of this book into super-sexy bite sizes, so you can choose your own adventure. Begin there, but let your desires wander. Pick one or more options from each section, put them together, and show your partner what you want.

Finding the Sensation You Want

As you read through the positions and determine which ones turn you on, think about the sensations you enjoy the most. A few specific sensations to consider:

GRIND Do you enjoy the body-on-body sensation of rubbing, pressure, friction, and pounding? Explore positions that include grinding, depth of penetration, and a lot of contact with all your awesome parts.

DEPTH Do you like to feel your bodies close together, your partner deep inside of you, or all of your cock or member being caressed and covered? If you're into feeling depth, look for positions that offer physical closeness, so you and your partner can both have the opportunity to go as deep as feels good.

FULLNESS Are you into feeling "filled up" or imagining that you are filling your partner up? That sensation can be incredibly erotic, exciting in its overwhelmingness, and an all-encompassing moment between the two of you. Look for positions that bring your bodies close together with the legs of the receiving partner closed or crossed. This will stimulate the feelings of tightness, fullness, and closeness that can feel so good.

THE IN-AND-OUT Love the stroke? Many nerve endings are located around the vaginal opening and in the sensitive labia and also in the opening of the anus. This is why penetration alone can be one of the most pleasurable elements of sex. To focus on this sensation and explore it further, look for positions with more separation and a bit more body distance, so you can play with shallow penetration and a longer stroke that is concentrated right around the opening of your partner's vagina or anus.

ANGLE Excited by working the G-spot or exploring all the hot buttons of both bodies? Look at the positions offering tilt and unique body angles, where your bodies are shifted from direct connection to somewhat off-center, above and below, sideways, and from-behind action. Play with the different heights of your hips and pelvises, and try shifting your hips and tailbones up and down in these positions to discover what button gets "pressed" and where.

CHAPTER 4

Intimate Sex Positions

INTIMACY IS A WORD FREQUENTLY USED WHEN DISCUSSING WHAT YOU WANT FROM YOUR RELATIONSHIPS with one another. But what is "intimate," exactly? It is a physical, energetic feeling of closeness and connection. It is awareness of your partner's presence, the feeling of being seen and met by them, and the knowledge that you understand them on a deep, emotional level. Intimacy is a presence and togetherness that allows you to relax and just be yourselves . . . and alleviates the need to explain or justify yourselves and your needs to each other.

The sex positions presented in this chapter are embracing, face-to-face, sincere, and focused, fostering body-to-body affinity so you can really connect to each other's energy. Intimate positions are positions for when you want to love and feel loved by your sexual partner, and they are great when you are looking to deepen your sync with each other or just to get back to feeling connected in those times when things have felt "off." These positions function best in locations where you are most comfortable and able to relax.

When you're in the mood for **INTIMATE SEX**, reach out to your partner like this:

1 START WITH SOME SEXY WORDS...

- "I feel so close to you."
- "I want to be close to you."
- "I want to connect with you."
- "You're so beautiful."
- "Let's get closer."
- "Let's just be together and touch each other."
- "I want to be naked with you."

- "Show me how you like to be touched."
- "Let's turn each other on."
- "It feels really good to be with you."
- "I love you."
- "Let's take our time tonight."
- "Let's cuddle."
- "I want to feel all of your body."
- "I love feeling you respond to me."

2 NEXT, REACH OUT AND TOUCH YOUR PARTNER...

- Tell your partner what feels delicious about being close to them and what you love about their body.
- Reach out and stroke your partner's hand and arm as they are talking.
- Enfold them in a hug, and hold them there longer than usual.
- Stroke the side of their face, and brush a piece of hair away from their face.
- Rub their back.
- Put your hand on the small of their back when they walk with you or when you're talking.
- Make eye contact and share your desire through your eyes.

- Cuddle close to them on the couch or when you're sitting next to one another.
- Lay your partner's head in your lap, and run your fingers through their hair.
- Press your body into their back and feel their warmth.
- Hold each other's hands.
- When you're together in a quiet moment, see if you can gently sync your breath to theirs.
- Take a bath or shower together.
- Watch your partner getting dressed or undressed, and really pay close attention.

- Give each other a slow massage that focuses on feeling each other's skin and muscles.

- Write down a moment in your day when you are thinking about them, and give them this piece of paper the next time you see them.

3 FINALLY, GET DOWN TO BUSINESS!

THE MISSIONARY PUSH-UP
(page 56)

THE IN-BETWEEN
(page 58)

SPOONS
(page 60)

THE KNEELING MISSIONARY
(page 62)

THE TANGLE
(page 64)

THE MISSIONARY FLIP
(page 66)

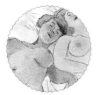

MUTUAL MASTURBATION
(page 68)

THE SEXY BACK
(page 70)

The Missionary Push-Up

KISSING • EYE CONTACT

"In *Samputa* your legs lie along hers, caressing their whole length from toes to thighs."

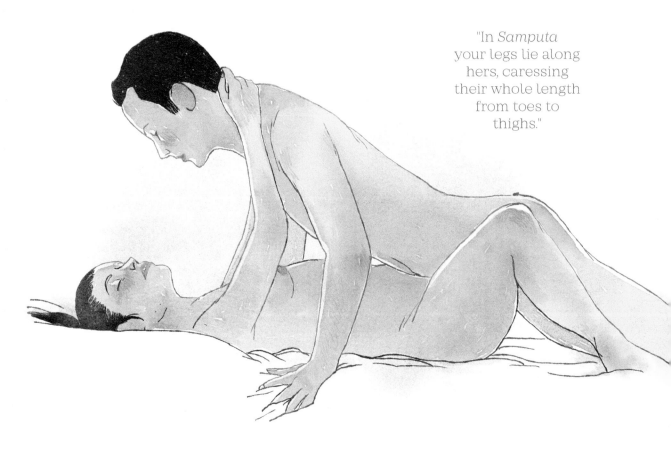

The Missionary Push-Up

VARIATION ON THE SAMPUTA POSITION (सम्पुट)

DESCRIPTION The Missionary Push-Up is dedicated to all those who love the Missionary position. Missionary is hands-down the world's most common sexual position, and for good reason: It provides lots of closeness and body contact as well as different levels of penetration. For those looking for a little something new, this variation adds some athleticism to the closeness and plays with distance and eye contact for maximum effect.

INSTRUCTIONS As with regular Missionary, finding a comfortable spot for the receiving partner is ideal; a bed, couch, or even soft rug on the floor works well. If you're going into this position wanting deeper penetration, make sure the receiving partner is lying on a firmer surface. First the receiving partner lies down on their back, and then the giving partner slides between their legs, bringing a hand to either side of their partner's body in a push-up and connecting in penetration.

Maybe you've heard of a similar position called CAT (Coital Alignment Technique). The Missionary Push-Up is different in that the giver's body is farther up, and when they lower their body their head goes to one side, putting both partners cheek-to-cheek. Instead of being chest to chest, the giver's chest is near the receiver's shoulders. Have the receiver bend her legs about 45 degrees to tilt her hips upward. This causes the base of the giver's shaft to maintain constant contact with her clitoris.

WHY YOU'LL LOVE IT While the traditional Missionary position is great for body contact, the Missionary Push-Up position allows for deeper penetration, more range of movement, and greater eye contact. The higher position of the giver's upper body creates space for deeper hip movement and thrust, and the closeness of both bodies produces a strong charge from hips to toes, rubbing and caressing, legs against legs, moving in and out. This position is particularly great for partners of different heights and weights, as the smaller partner can be on the bottom where they won't need to support the whole of their partner's weight or feel as if they are lost in the position.

DIFFICULTY ●●○○○ for the giving partner, ●○○○○ for the receiving partner

One of the best aspects of this position is the ability to connect, so make the most of locking eyes, listening to one another's breath, and allowing your partner to see just how good you feel. This is a great position to use when you are working on deepening and connecting to your own pleasure and physical sensations.

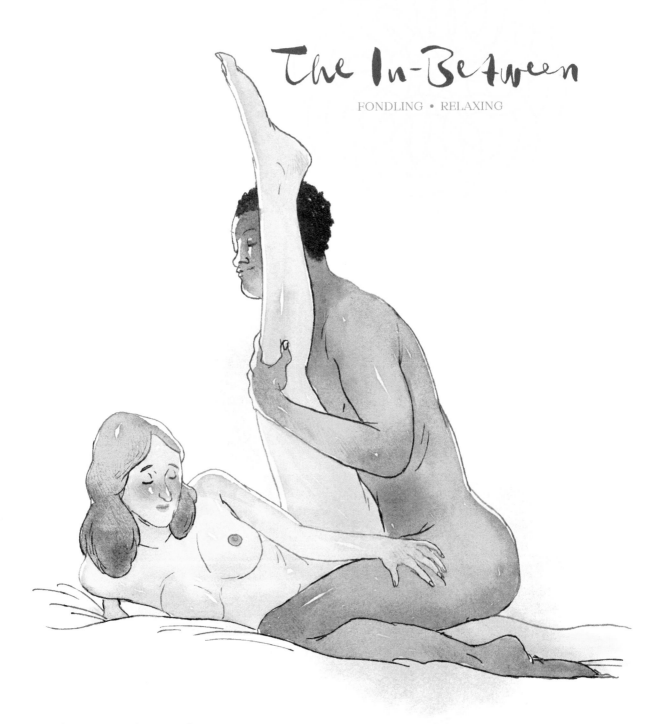

The In-Between

FONDLING • RELAXING

The In-Between

DESCRIPTION A position for those who love body connection and seek to explore both relaxation and depth of penetration. The In-Between offers connection through eye contact and touching, while allowing both partners to drop into their pleasure, reach deep into their enjoyment, and climb to orgasm.

INSTRUCTIONS The receiving partner lies down on a soft surface that provides gentle support, such as a bed or couch, and rolls over to their preferred side, lifting their top leg into the air. The giving partner then comes in on their knees, gently straddling their partner's bottom and extended leg, and moving into penetration between their partner's legs. The giving partner can then allow their receiving partner's top leg to rest on their chest, or use it to control depth and the force and speed of the action.

WHY YOU'LL LOVE IT Literally getting in between, this position brings you super close, but like some of the other intimate positions, it allows for plenty of eye contact and physical control. Each of you can drop into your own bodies and still feel connected. Great for penetration, the openness of the receiving partner's legs lets the giving partner find a depth and speed that feels good for both of you. When the receiving partner has open hips, this position leads to deeper penetration; when their hips are tighter, it allows for slow, controlled, gentler penetration. This position also offers a solid base for both partners, leaving your hands free for all kinds of grabbing, caressing, and exploring, both of your own and each other's bodies.

DIFFICULTY ●○○○○ for both partners

Finding this position less intense than you like? Try having the receiving partner angle their body from their side to their back, and see how this shift engages different parts of both of your bodies, allowing the receiver and giver access to their most turned-on parts.

Spoons

RELAXING · FONDLING

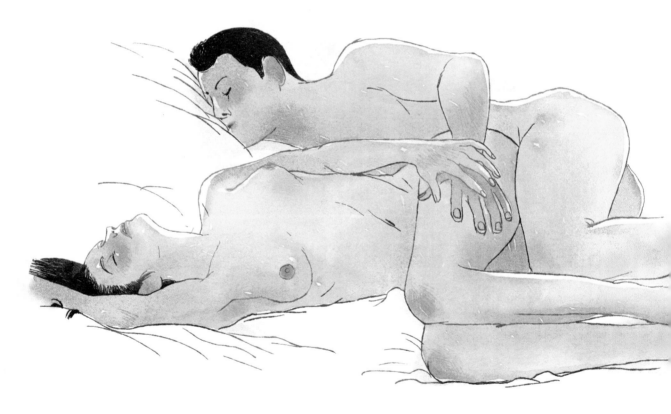

Spoons

DESCRIPTION Another classic that's one of the great intimate sex positions to explore, both as a go-to and one for making a gentle and sensual move on your partner. Because Spoons starts out with one partner behind the other, it's great for morning sex and for getting things moving in a sexy direction when you're cuddling and lying together.

INSTRUCTIONS Most of us are familiar with spooning, and this position takes it further to include penetration, possible reach-around, and plenty of moments to enjoy each other's bodies, butts, breasts, backs, and legs. Start out with one partner lying comfortably on their side. The giving partner then moves in behind so they are also lying on their side in the same position, their body "spooning" to cradle their partner, their front pressed up against their partner's back. In this position, enjoy feeling your partner's body pressed up against you, and see how you are both able to reach around from behind to caress each other. If you want to explore penetration, experiment with the angles at which you can touch and find entry. Either partner can bend at the waist or angle their body to find depth and stroke of penetration.

WHY YOU'LL LOVE IT Since spooning is a common sleeping position for many couples, it feels very natural and intimate in its sexual form. The relaxed position allows for your arms to do a whole lot of reaching and your hands to wander in all sorts of sexy ways: around, below, between. While this position doesn't allow for much eye contact, the giving partner will have a super-sexy view of some buns—this position is a butt lover's paradise. For the receiving partner, you'll notice how hot it feels to have your partner pressed up behind you and how this position allows you to feel their breath and enjoy their sexy words in your ear. Truly connective, this is a great position for a lazy, cozy day, or when you simply want to feel close.

DIFFICULTY ●○○○○ for both partners

Not getting enough penetration, or having trouble navigating your different heights? Try having the receiving partner lift their top leg and letting the giving partner move down and slide a bit more in between the receiver's legs. You may also want to try shifting so that your bodies form an X rather than a spooning shape, but allow yourselves to play and experiment in this position so that you both find your way to maximum pleasure.

The Kneeling Missionary

KISSING • SEXY VIEW

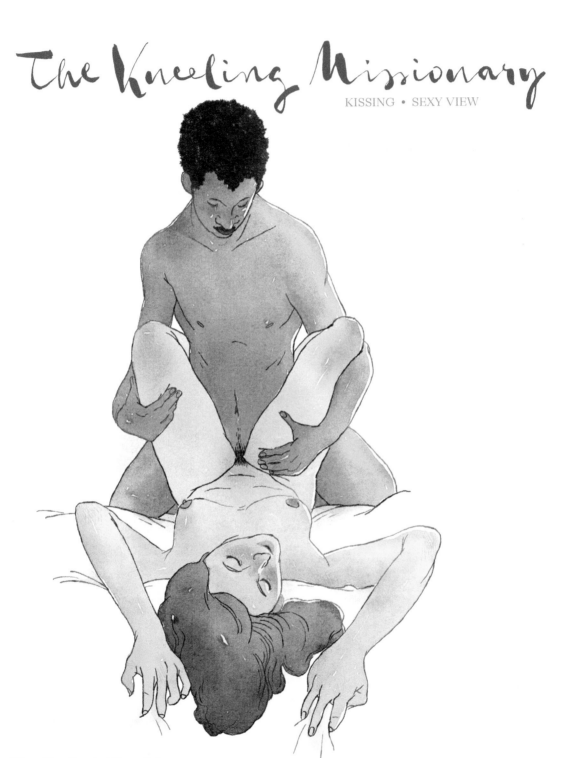

The Kneeling Missionary

DESCRIPTION This is another intimate position in which kneeling creates opportunities for comfort, closeness, and connection, as well as control in the depth and speed of penetration. Focusing on eye contact and playing with physical closeness and distance, this position gives both partners a chance to communicate what they like and find a pace and rhythm that works for both giver and receiver.

INSTRUCTIONS To begin, the giving partner kneels on a soft surface with their knees spaced out a bit. The receiving partner then lies on their back with their legs on either side of the kneeling partner's legs, then slides forward toward their partner, draping their legs over their partner's. In this beginning moment, there is a lot of full frontal and moments for access to each other's bodies, which is great for foreplay. Once you are both ready, the giving partner lifts up the receiving partner's hips and then controls the depth and thrust by moving up and down and pushing their own hips into those of their partner.

WHY YOU'LL LOVE IT This position falls under the intimate category because it offers a ton of full-on contact while providing moments for connection. The angle of your bodies as they connect makes for fun play with depth and thrust, as you touch and tease one another before you get into full penetrative sex. Folks with clitorises will love it because it gives them a chance to touch and be touched openly. Receiving partners will also love the feeling of being lifted by the strength of their giving partner, while both of you will enjoy being able to see each other's turn-on. In addition, this is a great position to explore G-spot stimulation and to discover how grinding increases your excitement.

DIFFICULTY ●○○○○ for the receiving partner, ●●○○○ for the giving partner

Feel like all the control is in the giving partner's hands? This move is the perfect opportunity for the receiving partner to focus on their body, offering the giving partner a little show of self-touch and seeing how much that gets them excited. Just ping-pong that hot energy back and forth!

The Tangle

FEELING CONNECTED • KISSING

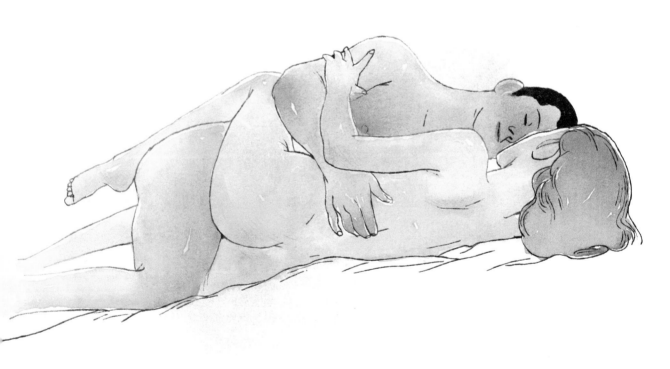

The Tangle

DESCRIPTION For those who love Spoons (page 60) and the Missionary position and want a little bit of each for an intimate moment. In this position, your bodies are wrapped together in a full-frontal variation on spooning, allowing you to move and grind and discover how you fit together best. Great for making the transition from cuddling to slowly grinding to penetration, this position is all about rolling around with one another, grabbing, holding, and touching in ways that feel amazing and bring you deeper into powerful energetic intimacy.

INSTRUCTIONS One of the terrific things about this position is that you can get into it while cuddling, kissing, or just having a mellow moment together. It's also great to use as a bridge when moving from one position to another. Begin by lying down facing one another, each of you on your side. In this position, both partners are giving and receiving, so begin by draping arms across one another, grabbing backs and butts, and touching each other's faces. Move into it more deeply by having one partner bring their leg in between the other's legs, and continue intertwining legs so you are able to grind and eventually find your way to penetration. As you maintain your physical closeness throughout this position, each of you may want to try rolling on top or shifting your weight to enjoy it even more.

WHY YOU'LL LOVE IT One word? Closeness. Like many of the other positions in this section, this one is all about intimacy and feeling each other's skin and bodies to the utmost. Because this position feels like wrestling, you may notice how quickly the energy gets ramped up. Allow it to take you to greater intensity, and play with pace to see what you enjoy the most. While penetration is possible in this position, the main event is your intertwining, grinding, and overall contact. You will enjoy experimenting with your degree of turn-on and what you want to get from this position, so feel the flow as you use it to take you from one moment into the next.

DIFFICULTY ●○○○○ for both partners

Folks with clits, try seeing how the grind of a leg between yours feels great, and play with gripping and relaxing your legs during penetration to change up the feel of sex for both of you.

The Missionary Flip

FONDLING • SEXY VIEW

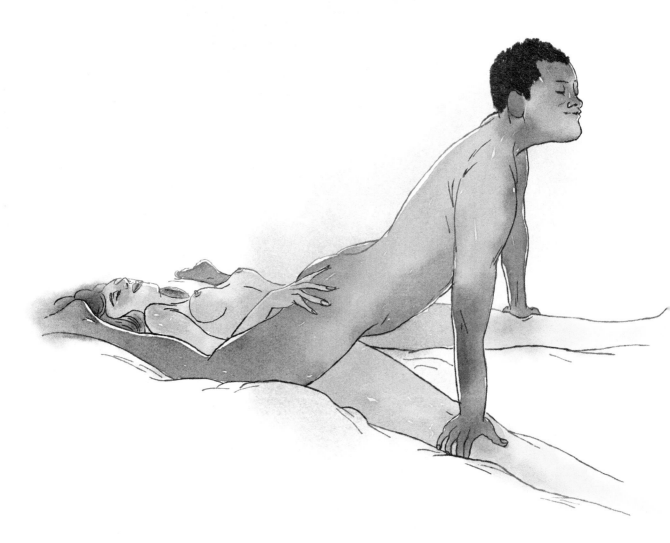

The Missionary Flip

DESCRIPTION This position takes a go-to classic and literally flips it around so you can see what other placements of your body can do to charge arousal, fulfill great penetration, and give you new views to explore. While this position is incredibly intimate, it will push you gently out of your comfort zone, so try it when you're feeling playful and seeking closeness with a twist.

INSTRUCTIONS For this position, you want to make sure you have one or two firm pillows and a soft resting place that's not too squishy—lying on a sheeted mattress or on a soft blanket on the floor is perfect. The receiving partner lies down on the floor with one or two pillows beneath their hips and lower back. The giving partner then lies on top, facing the opposite direction toward legs and feet, with belly down. When in position, the partner below has great access to their partner above's buns, and the partner on top has their head down toward their receiving partner's feet.

If you're using this position for penetration, make sure the penetrating partner is on top. The receiving partner can spread their legs to allow the top partner's upper body to rest on the floor between their legs. Alternatively, if you want to experiment with depth and squeeze, the bottom partner can try closing their legs and supporting their partner's body length and weight with their thighs and shins.

WHY YOU'LL LOVE IT There is so much fun to be had in this position! Simply by reversing the usual perspective on one another's bodies, you will get to explore newness and how exciting it feels to be in full body contact with different parts of one another. For the partner on top, this may encourage much more touching for your butt than you have gotten in a while, and you will feel how much fun that is for your partner beneath you. For the partner below, notice how it feels to support your partner's weight and to be physically close without eye contact. While penetration is one aspect of this position, notice that it's not set up for that to be the most important part, and experiment with how you can get closer, grind on one another, and enjoy slight penetration while rocking and flowing and moving together.

DIFFICULTY ●○○○○ for the receiving partner, ●●○○○ for the giving partner

---

Looking for a great transition from this position to the next? Try having the partner on top back it up and bring their hips and parts over the receiver's face in a sexy tease. Want to take it to a whole new level? Have the partner on top suck on the bottom partner's toes, giving their feet a squeeze, and playing with sensations in the legs and feet.

Mutual Masturbation

KISSING • TURN-ON

Mutual Masturbation

DESCRIPTION One of the most common complaints I hear from clients is, "We want to connect, but sometimes we are just too tired." This is the position I recommend for low-energy nights, when you can each take care of yourself and focus on your own pleasure while sharing that next to your partner.

INSTRUCTIONS Begin on a bed or comfortable surface, in a spot where each of you can extend your legs. You're going to lie side by side, on your backs, eyes to the ceiling, your ears next to one another, and the top of one of your heads in the crook of the other's shoulder and neck. You will feel like your mouths are close and every noise you make can be heard by your partner. This is a crucial part of this position. As you touch yourself, allow your noises to flow out of you; simultaneously, notice the sounds of your partner and how they turn you on. You will notice that you can hear and feel your partner's strong energy but not see much of what they are doing. This little bit of sensory deprivation will make you curious and help play up the energy. Find you can't take it? Jump their bones! There's that energy for sex you didn't think you had!

WHY YOU'LL LOVE IT This position is unconventional in terms of the amount of distance between your bodies, but it is a great way to focus on listening, being together, and feeling each other's energy. Never masturbated in front of your partner? This is the perfect beginning pose because they will be able to hear and enjoy how good things feel for you without you feeling watched. Hearing breath and moans and feeling energy build is a huge turn-on, and getting yourself off, feeling the kind of touch you want in that moment, can be very satisfying and empowering.

DIFFICULTY ●○○○○ for both partners

 Notice how allowing yourself to feel pleasure impacts your partner; this can be a great exercise in letting your sexual energy flow without shame.

The Sexy Back

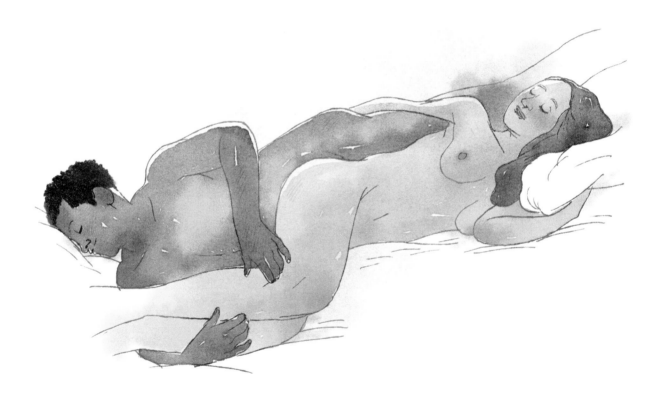

The Sexy Back

DESCRIPTION Do you love the Spoons position (page 60) but hate that you don't get to see much of your partner enjoying themselves and enjoying you? This flip variation on spooning lets both of you watch and enjoy while still getting the benefits of rear entry plus a lot of butt appreciation. Great for days when you're feeling less energetic, this one can be entered into slowly and casually and can work with both of you propped up on an elbow or lying on your side—think of it as lazy-bed-day-turns-hot with lots of fondling, grinding, and penetration.

INSTRUCTIONS Start with your heads at opposite ends of a bed or couch, on the floor, or on a soft blanket. The receiving partner lies on one side, legs outstretched and relaxed. The giving partner moves in, their pelvis to their receiving partner's butt, head down by their feet so you both can look at one another. Begin with some great butt massage, grinding your hips, pelvis, and butt into one another to charge the energy, and feel yourselves get more and more turned on. When you feel ready, let penetration happen slowly between pressed-together legs, squeezing tight, or have the receiving partner open their top leg to drape over their bottom leg, gently tilting their buns away from the giving partner.

WHY YOU'LL LOVE IT If you love the closeness of spooning, this position has a ton to offer with the added bonus of eye contact, relaxed body position, and a whole lot of opportunity for back and butt rubbing—not to mention booty appreciation! With your legs outstretched, play with the tightness and grip of penetration, and experiment with bending your body at the waist to get deeper penetration or backing up your butt to intensify the grind. You can steady yourself and increase control by propping yourself up on one elbow, or simply relax into it and enjoy the ride. Giving partners have a lot of body to enjoy, and receiving partners will experience how good the closeness feels from behind.

DIFFICULTY ●●○○○ for both partners

Love this position? Let both of your bodies roll over onto your bellies, and see how you can continue the penetration from there. It may be a challenge, but it creates a whole new position to explore!

CHAPTER 5

Energetic Sex Positions

YOU KNOW THAT SURGE OF ENERGY YOU FEEL IN YOUR BODY AT ALL DIFFERENT TIMES, LIKE FIRST thing in the morning, after a great workout, or during an exciting moment? That energetic feeling can often move right into powerful sexual desire, and the positions in this chapter are designed to harness the power of those occasions. Some of the most exciting sexual experiences can be ones where you wrestle, grab, move expansively and athletically, and find yourself breathing heavily, heart racing and muscles taut. When a physical situation requires your body to rise to the occasion or respond to it, the sensations that result are intense and can be truly sensational.

These sex positions are energetic, rigorous, and athletic for both partners. Energetic positions are great for when you're feeling in the mood to get wild and push beyond what feels like your usual routine. They are positions that send you deeper into awareness of your body by asking you to push yourself. Just like an exercise class, these energetic positions will require effort. They challenge you on a physical level and make you sweat, and they reward you with new perspectives on your body and how to "get physical" with your partner.

When you're in the mood for **ENERGETIC SEX**, reach out to your partner like this:

1 START WITH SOME SEXY WORDS...

- "Let's try something new."
- "I want to get physical with you."
- "Let's get wild and crazy tonight."
- "I have a sexy surprise for you."
- "I wanna ragdoll you around a little."
- "I'm feeling so on fire to be with you."
- "I'm feeling extra energetic, let's romp."
- "Getting out sexual energy with you is my favorite."
- "Come here and let me show you what this feels like."

- "You make my body go crazy."
- "I want us to push ourselves and each other."
- "Fuck the gym, let's get sweaty right here."
- "I want to see all that your body can do."
- "It really turns me on when we do new things together."
- "Watching you push yourself gets me off."

2 NEXT, REACH OUT AND TOUCH YOUR PARTNER...

- Stretch with your partner, allowing yourself to get turned on by their body.
- Grab your partner's booty, and squeeze your favorite parts. Notice the thrill you get.
- Initiate sex right where you are; take it to the floor, the wall, the nearest piece of furniture. Don't focus on comfort, go for grabbing the moment.
- Show your partner your excited energy. Let them see you full of buzzy vibes to get sexy.
- Touch your partner's body as if it's a playground just for you.

- Take an exercise class with your partner, and continue it right into the locker room, car, living room, or bedroom.
- Grab your partner right when they get home from the gym. To hell with the sweat! You're just going to get sweatier anyway!
- Chase your partner playfully, and when you catch them, hold on tight! A little tension can get things going.
- Reach out and pull your partner toward you. Even from a distance, gather their energy to you.

- Have a strong partner? Jump on for a piggyback ride, and let your giggles lead you into kissing and grabbing their neck and body.

- When you masturbate, get about halfway to your orgasm, then go get your partner for a romp around. Use the energy you've built to keep exploring.

- Try moving each other's bodies around. Push and shove a little, and see how it feels to get physical.

3 FINALLY, GET DOWN TO BUSINESS!

THE PLOW
(page 76)

THE SEX SWING
(page 78)

THE UNDERCARRIAGE
(page 80)

THE LEG UP
(page 82)

THE THIGH RIDER
(page 84)

THE FULL FRONTAL
(page 86)

THE SLINKY
(page 88)

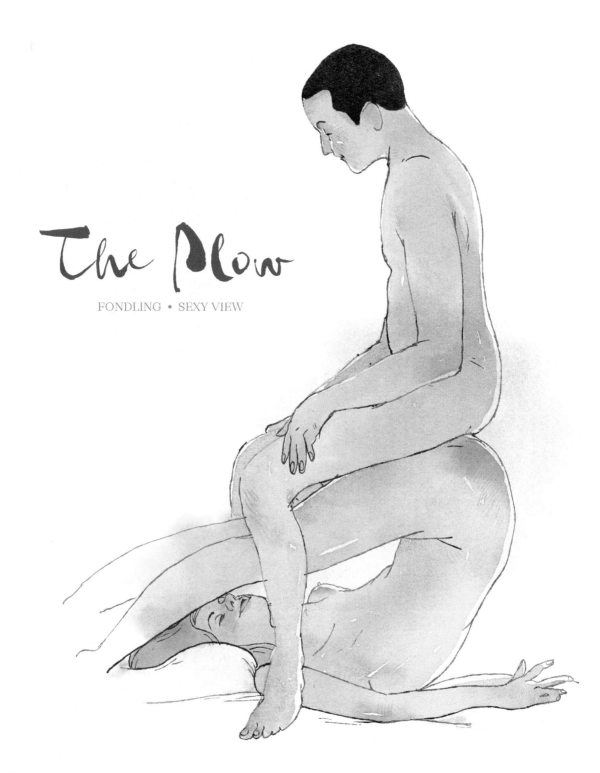

The Plow

FONDLING • SEXY VIEW

The Plow

DESCRIPTION The Plow is designed for maximum access and penetration, as well as an incredibly hot view of both partners' bodies from above and below. Once you get the hang of it, feel free to experiment with leg and hand positions.

INSTRUCTIONS Start out by finding a bed, couch, or large, low chair. The person moving into the bottom position sits on the bed or couch with their back to the edge. Moving slowly, and getting help from their partner, they slide off the edge of the bed and onto the floor, until they are resting on their shoulders with their lower back balanced vertically up on the side of the bed or couch. Legs can go in a variety of positions: together and over your head with toes reaching for the floor behind you, spread wide into a *V* and bent at the knees, or knees pulled into the chest in a crouch.

The partner on top then straddles their receiving partner's body, legs on either side of their butt and legs. The partner on top then has many choices for how they get going; bending forward using their mouth, reaching down and using fingers, or penetrating their partner with their cock by squatting and using their thigh muscles to move in and out of their partner.

WHY YOU'LL LOVE IT This position is high energy and extra erotic. The partner on the bottom is using a lot of physical control to hold their position and offer their body up to their straddling partner above. This provides extra-deep penetration and allows for an almost endless number of possibilities for playing with all kinds of sex acts.

The receiving partner will love experiencing the strength of their partner, and the giving partner will love the access they have to view their partner below in such an open position.

Both partners have their hands free in this position, so figuring out how you want to support yourself best and touch your partner can be a fun challenge. There are also fun ways to experiment with leaning forward and back.

DIFFICULTY ●●●○○ for the standing partner, ●●●●● for the partner below

---

For the partner on the bottom, it can feel like you get compressed and that it's hard to take a deep breath. Don't let the shortness of breath take you out of your body; see if you can use the shorter breaths to fire that excitement you get from seeing your partner so tall above you. Positions that make you feel vulnerable can be scary, but pay attention to what you like about feeling smaller or exposed, and let the position take you to unexplored places in your body.

The Sex Swing

CARDIO • EYE CONTACT

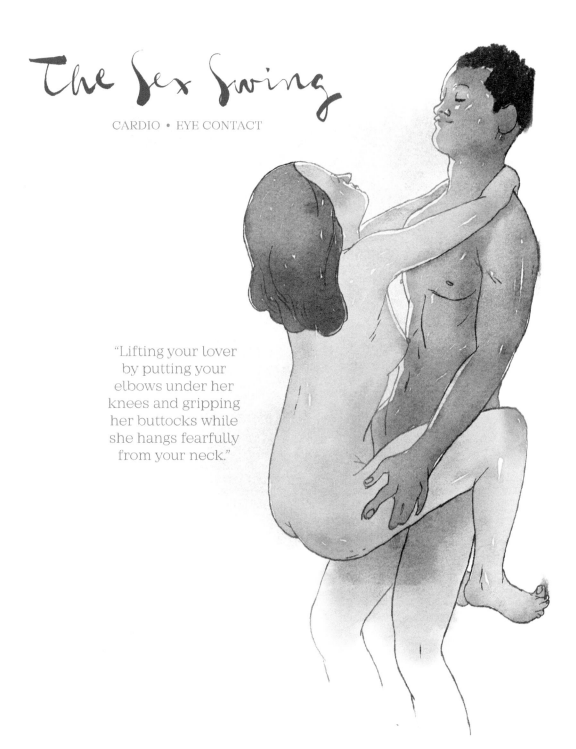

"Lifting your lover by putting your elbows under her knees and gripping her buttocks while she hangs fearfully from your neck."

The Sex Swing

JANUKURPARA (जानु कूर्पर)

DESCRIPTION This is a truly acrobatic and exciting position that will give you a thrill. The *Kama Sutra* recommends standing and swinging positions for when you want to fan the sexual flames of your relationship, and it points out how trying something physically challenging during sex brings two people closer, allowing them to feel proud when they find a new position that is both fun and successful.

INSTRUCTIONS The standing partner stands, legs spread, back against a wall, and bends in a squat to link their arms around the back of their partner's knees. The hanging partner then links their arms around the standing partner's neck and brings their knees to their chest as their partner lifts them from behind the knees.

Once off the ground, the hanging partner can push their feet against the wall while both partners find their way to penetration. Having established a good connection, the hanging partner can pump their legs to grind and bounce on and off of their partner. The standing partner can clasp their hands beneath their partner's knees or grab handfuls of buns.

WHY YOU'LL LOVE IT Being supported by a standing partner can be an incredibly energetic experience—you'll feel both weightless and held at the same time. The hanging partner will feel a bit like a sexy ragdoll and enjoy the sense of how their body can control penetration through leg pumping and holding on more tightly or loosely to their partner's neck. Meanwhile, the standing partner can aim penetration wherever they want and control the height of their swinging partner as well as how close they hold them to their own body. While this position does require a lot of muscle strength, you'll be fired up by all that blood pumping through your muscles and the opportunity to feel ultra-strong and in control.

Energetic positions are the ones you can really lose yourself in with abandon. Once you've reached a good flow for penetration, let yourself really get going— speed it up or slow it down to see what feels best.

DIFFICULTY ●●●●● for the hanging partner, ●●●●○ for the standing partner

---

Love this one but want more stability and deeper, harder penetration? Turn the position around so the hanging partner has their back against the wall. Have the standing partner move their hands to the hanging partner's buns and really push up against them, feeling how you can get deeper while still appreciating your partner hanging wild around your neck.

The Undercarriage

ENERGIZING • SEXY VIEW

"She stands on palms and feet, you stand behind her and lift one of her feet to your shoulder, then enjoying *'Traivikrama.'*"

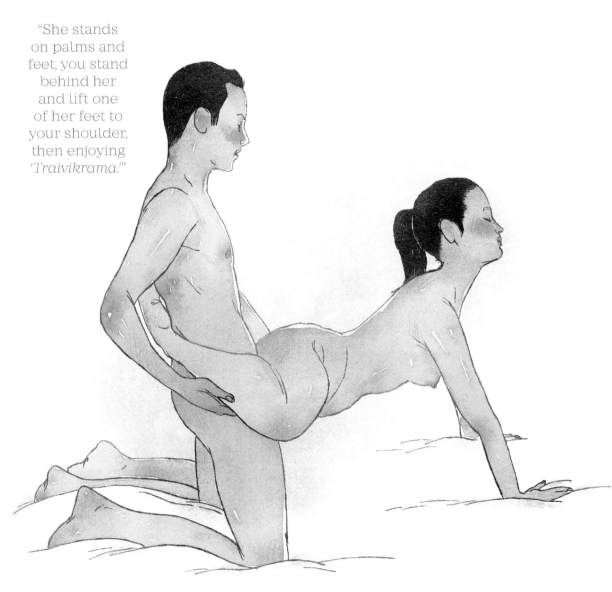

The Undercarriage

TRAIVIKRAMA (त्रैविक्रम)

DESCRIPTION Adventurous and crazy fun to get into, this position is excellent for finding new rhythms and exploring how your bodies connect. Since it's a standing position, it can make you feel strong and fully in your body. It's also seductive and exposing in ways that make for great flashbacks to this position later on. This position will be extra entertaining for those who are more flexible, but it can be modified with a more stable bottom position.

INSTRUCTIONS The receiving partner starts out standing with their feet spaced shoulder width apart, bending forward at the waist to place their palms flat in front of them on the floor to create a stable base. The giving partner then moves up behind their receiving partner and gently, but with good support, moves one of their partner's legs out sideways, bringing it up, back, and around their own waist, providing support by positioning their arm underneath their partner's extended leg. If the receiving partner is very flexible, try moving toward a standing split, resting their upstretched leg on their partner's chest, or hooking their foot onto their partner's shoulder.

WHY YOU'LL LOVE IT Not only is this position awesome for deep penetration, but it also allows your bodies to find a good mutual flow, charging up your sexual energy. The bottom partner creates most of the stability in this position, and the giving partner dials the intensity up or down, depending on the speed of their thrusts and the position of their body.

The demanding nature of this position will drive concentration, deep body awareness, and breathing that will help you maintain your stability and stoke your fire and arousal. Once you find your flow and let yourself just go with it, this position can be absolutely incredible.

DIFFICULTY ● ● ● ● ● for both partners

Struggling with stability in this position? Try having the bottom partner position their body in front of a wall or near the bed so they can press their palms flat on the floor against a steady block to keep from sliding forward. Still looking for a change that can help you relax a bit? Take this position down to all fours, still keeping one leg up and wrapped around your partner's waist or hanging from their shoulder. See if this helps you feel more pleasure, and notice how your breath changes. Keep the more athletic version in your repertoire, but let yourself come to your knees when you want to bring the energy down a notch or two.

The Leg Up

CARDIO • KISSING

The Leg Up

DESCRIPTION This position is ideal for partners with flexible legs and open hips and offers variations so you can get in where you fit in and still enjoy maximum body contact. It's designed for maximum erotic energy and feels exciting and new.

INSTRUCTIONS Begin with both partners standing, pressed against one another, chest to chest. The giving partner reaches down and brings one of their partner's legs up to rest on their shoulder while wrapping their arms around their partner's back, supporting that lifted leg under the buttock. The partner with their leg up wraps their arms around the giving partner's neck. The receiving partner will be pinned against the giving partner, who controls most of the action.

WHY YOU'LL LOVE IT While the receiving partner does need to be flexible to get into this position, having their body held up like this can feel incredible and be great for full-body contact and penetration. Experiment with standing on flat feet or tiptoes. Even if this position doesn't feel possible for very long, it can be great to let yourself enjoy the restraint and athletic, intense sensation for even a short time. The giving partner will love the feeling of strength and the access it gives them to their partner's body, as well as the control it provides over thrust.

Variations can also be fun to explore: Try having the lifted-leg partner lean against a wall and encourage them to bend the raised leg at the knee to see if that helps with the split stretch occurring in the hip and groin. The focus of this position is on the super-sexy energy that comes from pushing physical limits, rather than the need to execute the pose absolutely perfectly.

DIFFICULTY ●●●○○ for the giving partner, ●●●●● for the receiving partner

---

Getting tired? Try having the receiving partner drop their leg around the giving partner's waist so they can grab both of their partner's butt cheeks and really savor the kissing, neck biting, and other possibilities of total closeness.

The Thigh Rider

FONDLING • GRINDING

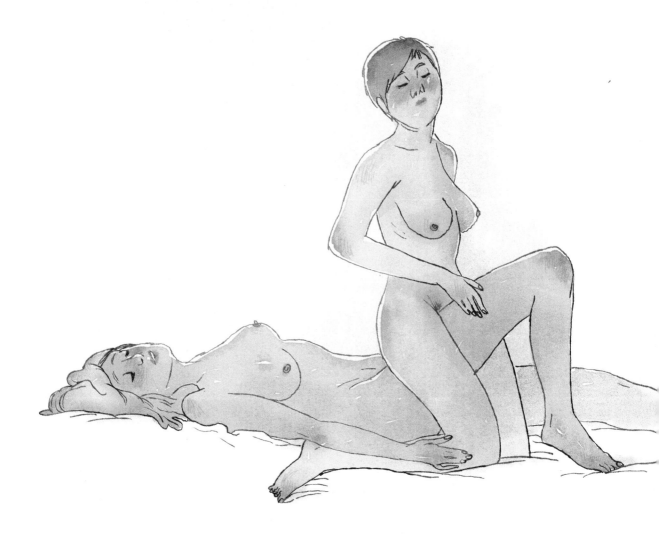

The Thigh Rider

DESCRIPTION I often hear clients with pussies complain that there aren't enough sexual positions that focus on clitoral stimulation. While reverse cowgirl is a classic, it can be limiting for some bodies. I designed the Thigh Rider to have variable aspects that will allow the partner on top to try a few different physical locations to get off in a way they enjoy. Feel free to try this position with and without penetration, and experience the deepest pleasure you can find.

INSTRUCTIONS Since the pressure is really centered at the hips and butt where bodies can take a good deal of weight, give this one a try wherever you might be when the mood strikes. Start with one partner lying flat on their back, extending one leg and bending the other leg so the foot rests on the floor with their knee up. The other partner can then straddle or climb on, whatever way feels best, settling into penetration or just nestling in so their parts are right up against their partner's thigh.

WHY YOU'LL LOVE IT This position is intimate, connective, and all about the pleasure of the partner on top. The top partner can determine how to move their body and experiment with depth and penetration as they grind. They are also in a good position to play with self-touch and reach through their legs to fondle their partner's parts, too. The partner below gets an excellent view of their partner's buns moving as they grind and rock back and forth, and they, too, have a good opportunity to stroke and explore their own body. There is something for everyone in this position, and the connection comes through each of you dropping into your own pleasure simultaneously.

DIFFICULTY ●○○○○ for both partners

Close your eyes and notice how that varies your experience. Because you aren't looking at one another, this can be a great position for fantasizing, vocalizing your moans and how good things feel, and letting your sensations take over. Find it hard to keep your eyes closed? Try this one blindfolded.

The Full Frontal

EYE CONTACT • FONDLING

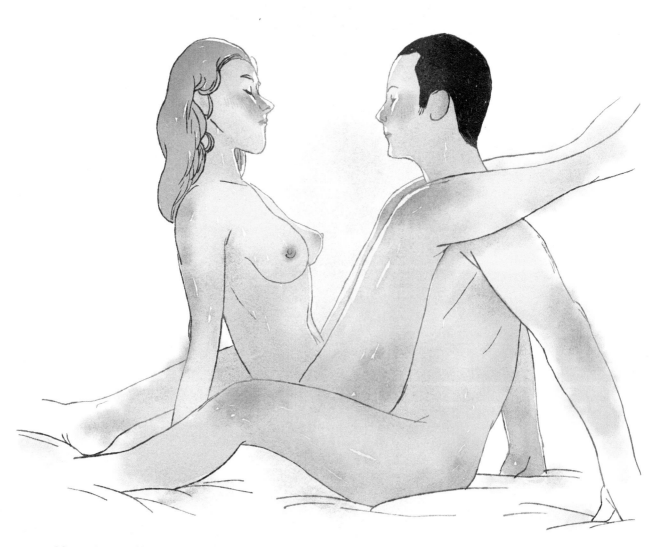

The Full Frontal

GRAMYA (ग्राम्य)

DESCRIPTION This position is great for penetration and can bring your bodies super close if you're flexible; if you're not very bendy, it still can be a lot of fun to see where your arms and legs can go. Approach this one in the spirit of connection and experimentation, and you'll find it has a lot to offer both of you.

INSTRUCTIONS Start with the giving partner propped up against the head of a bed, couch, or wall, and with their legs extended comfortably in front of them. If this feels uncomfortable, they can extend both arms behind them to hold their upper body upright.

The receiving partner then straddles the bottom partner, settling into penetration if desired. From there, using their hands as support, the top partner brings their legs up and onto the bottom partner's shoulders. Once the top partner has settled into place, they can experiment with using their planted hands and arm strength to move them in grinding and finding their flow. The partner on the bottom can also use their arms to push the top partner back and forth.

WHY YOU'LL LOVE IT Much like the other energetic positions, this one takes some work to get into, but at the same time it creates an opportunity to connect and bond in the challenge of finding how you fit together. Because of how folded together your bodies are in this position, it is great for penetration and for getting to see each other exposed and super turned on.

While this position can be difficult for making big movements, its athleticism comes in the holding and maintaining, rather than in hard thrusting. Focus on finding your rock and roll together, syncing your breathing, and experimenting with eye contact. The partner on top will love the feeling of being folded and the challenge of holding the position, while the partner on bottom will relish the sensation of the top partner moving into position and finding their pleasure in the grind and penetration. Focus on the fun here, and transition by letting the top partner's legs come down whenever they want.

DIFFICULTY ●○○○○ for the giving partner, ●●●○○ for the receiving partner

---

Not finding this position intense enough? Have the bottom partner use the support of the wall or furniture behind them to allow their arms to go free, and encourage them to try clasping their arms around their partner's back instead, really folding them into a sexy, tight package. With the top partner folded that securely, most of the flow of grind and penetration will come from the bottom partner.

The Slinky

CONTROL • FONDLING

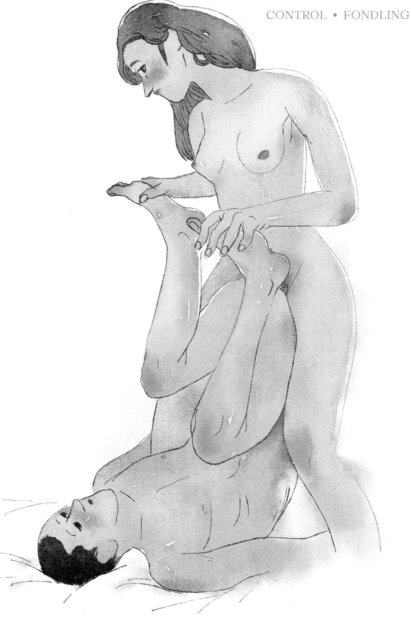

The Slinky

DESCRIPTION Feeling stuck in a rut? This position offers a silly and super-hot option for trying something new with your partner and can be great for bonding. While intercourse is a part of the position, it need not be the main event to make this position fun. Start out by following the instructions below, and allow your bodies to transition into different poses and configurations, discovering the heat and arousal as you go.

INSTRUCTIONS Find a very comfortable spot to try this one, the softer and squishier the better. The giving partner begins on their back with their legs folded up in the fetal position, slowly bringing their butt higher into the air. The receiving partner then straddles the bottom partner's butt and slowly moves down into a kneeling position, dropping into penetration or into a gentle grind.

The flow and movement of this position comes from the thigh strength of the partner below, as well as from the thigh strength of the straddling partner, who uses their legs to ground them and keep them from dropping all of their weight onto their partner. Once you feel settled into the position, experiment with using your arms to hold one another in place, or fondle and caress one another as you move. If you can't stay in the position for more than a few minutes, simply allow yourselves to flow into another one.

WHY YOU'LL LOVE IT This position is physically demanding but also incredibly fun and great for body exploration. If you're experimenting with penetration, the rolled-up position of the bottom partner enables you to go deep, and it can even be fun for trying anal sex. The bottom partner might enjoy the sensation of keeping their thighs together while their partner bounces on top of them, and the partner on top can take pleasure in the ride from above and the power of their partner's body below.

DIFFICULTY ● ● ● ● ● for both partners

Enjoying how wild and fun this position feels? Try it next to a piece of sturdy furniture that you can hold on to really get buck wild. Who needs a gym when your own bodies can serve as workout equipment?

CHAPTER 6

Powerful Sex Positions

FROM NEGOTIATIONS IN ADVANCE TO THE ENERGY EXCHANGE BEFORE, AFTER, AND DURING, power performs a huge role in sexual play. How do we feel powerful, who holds the power, and what turns us on about shifting power dynamics? Playing with power is one of the easiest ways to experiment with adding charge to your sexual relationship, and it is a topic clients are always especially curious to discuss. If you feel powerful in most parts of your lives, you may want to shift into a less commanding energy in sexual play or learn how to transfer that powerful energy from the rest of life into sex. If, on the other hand, you are the kind of person who doesn't identify with feeling powerful, you might want to explore ways to experience that feeling during intimacy.

These sex positions are carnal, aggressive, and dominating, immediately drawing your awareness to the power dynamic between you and your partner. These positions are great for experimentation and roleplay, as well as bringing in elements like bondage and impact play.

When you're in the mood for **POWERFUL SEX**, reach out to your partner like this:

1 START WITH SOME SEXY WORDS...

- "Come here."
- "I want to have my way with you."
- "You are so hot."
- "I need to have you right now."
- "I want to feel you submit to me."
- "I want to feel you overpower me."
- "I love it when you throw me down."
- "You are one sexy fuck."
- "Get aggressive with me."

- "I love feeling your dominance."
- "Make me feel your power."
- "Let's play harder tonight."
- "I want to get rough with you."
- "Let me take control."
- "I want you to take control."
- "Use my body for your pleasure."
- "I'm going to show you what I want."

2 NEXT, REACH OUT AND TOUCH YOUR PARTNER...

- Move toward your partner and push them up against a wall before kissing them.
- Push them up against the wall, then hold them there while you look up and down their body.
- Sneak up on your partner from behind, and bring a hand under their chin, gently tilting their head back.
- Reach over and run your hand down your partner's thigh, giving it a firm squeeze.
- Look at your partner like you want to take a huge bite out of them.
- Corner your partner in the bedroom, and kiss them down onto the bed.

- Tease and entice your partner by undressing where they can see just a little bit of you.
- Get down on all fours and crawl into the bedroom.
- Leave any of the toys or other items you want to play with out on the bed or where your partner can see them when they get home.
- Send your partner pictures of you biting your lip in excitement. Look for visual references of what you want and email or text them to your partner during the day.

- With one hand, grab your partner's hips from behind, then place your other hand on their back between their shoulders and gently press them forward.
- Grab your partner by the hair with your hands deep and all the way down to the roots, then squeeze your hands gently, being careful not to tug.
- When you're making out, tilt your partner's head back by nudging the bottom of their chin with your nose, and kiss them hungrily on the neck.
- Let your hands walk down your partner's body until you're on your knees in front of them, looking up.
- First make sure that your partner is okay with a little roughhousing, then take them down to the floor when it's unexpected and you're really feeling it.

3 FINALLY, GET DOWN TO BUSINESS!

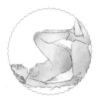

THE G HUNTER
(page 94)

THE FULL PRESS
(page 96)

THE GREAT WALL
(page 98)

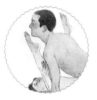

THE FOLD
(page 100)

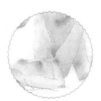

V FORCE
(page 102)

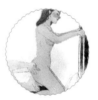

THE HIJACK
(page 104)

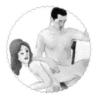

OVER THE KNEE
(page 106)

THE ARCH
(page 108)

The G Hunter

EYE CONTACT • CONTROL

"With the receiving partner lying on her back, you sit between her parted knees, raise them, hook her feet over your thighs, catch hold of her breasts, and enjoy her."

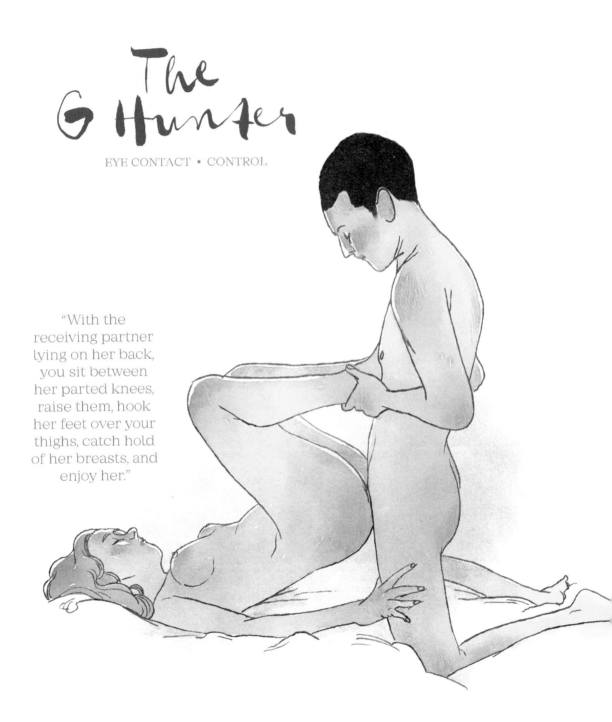

The G Hunter

A VARIATION ON MANMATHPRIYA (मन्मथप्रिय)

DESCRIPTION From the name alone, those interested in G-spot action and/or discovery can tell they are in for a lot of fun in this position. It belongs in the category of powerful positions because both partners can enjoy the closeness and power of their bodies held in tension, pressing back and forth. The bottom partner will notice how being folded up and small can feel both submissive and powerful, while the partner on top can explore their power through pressure and determining how much of their body is holding their partner down as they thrust and move.

INSTRUCTIONS Start out on a bed or other nice, soft surface. The receiving partner begins on their back, rolling their knees up to touch their chest and partially bringing up their butt as well. The giving partner then moves in so the receiving partner's butt is around their belly and chest level, and they gently roll into penetration and grinding by pushing down onto the receiving partner and then slowly pulling back and folding over their body.

The power of this position mostly rests with the partner on top, but the receiving partner may notice the strength of their thighs as soon as they begin to hold any of their partner's weight. The partner on top can either use their hands and arms as support or rest all of their weight on the bottom partner and use their hands for touching, caressing, and more powerful forms of physical communication.

WHY YOU'LL LOVE IT As in many other positions in which one or both partners are folded, the way your bodies fit together in this pose can be amazing for G-spot stimulation, experimenting with depth and pace of penetration, and focusing on closeness and energy exchange. Because this position is somewhat physically demanding, it will get your heart rate going and complicate your breath, which in turn will heighten your awareness of new sensations and experiences. Being so close to one another also allows for deep eye contact and experimenting with getting close and pushing away. With so many elements to play with, this is a position you can sustain and enjoy for quite a while.

DIFFICULTY ●●○○○ for the receiving partner, ●●●○○ for the giving partner

Does the receiving partner find the pressure on their legs too intense or need a break to breathe? Try transitioning into the In-Between (page 58) or Kneeling Missionary (page 60) and see if you prefer to stay in a more relaxed position for penetration.

The Full Press

FONDLING • FEELING CONNECTED

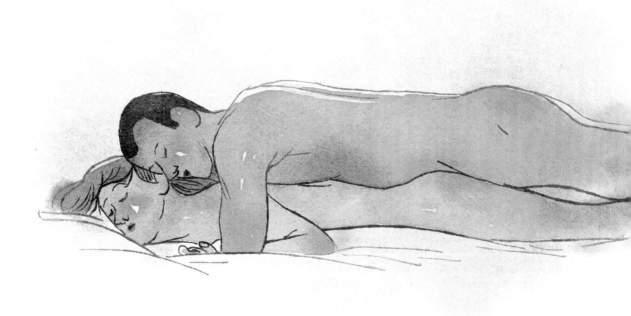

The Full Press

DESCRIPTION Incredibly close and powerful in its full-body contact, this position allows for experimentation with weight, dirty talk, body worship, touching, and all kinds of penetration. It's designed for those bun-loving folks out there who'd love nothing more than to see their partner's beautiful body stretched out—and to be able to touch them by laying their own body on top.

INSTRUCTIONS The receiving partner begins by lying down on their belly, head resting gently to one side and legs stretched out, thighs together. (You need not have a super-comfy surface for this one, but check in with your body as things progress, and see how pressure and weight are affecting you.) The giving partner then lies down on top of the receiving partner, fully stretched out, head up by their partner's ear. The giving partner stretches their legs open a bit and uses toes and hands as support on either side of their partner. Both partners work together to achieve penetration, noticing how it can take place between thighs or sliding along butt cheeks.

WHY YOU'LL LOVE IT While truly intimate and close in a warm and cozy way, this position is also ideal for playing with power. Consider it full-body bondage, as the receiving/bottom partner will be fully held down by their partner's weight. Depending on your bodies, penetration may be shallow or a bit deeper, but the closeness of thighs and the squeeze of limbs together will make for fun, tight, and soft spaces to explore and enjoy in new ways. Because this position is intense but also relaxed, you may find that you can stay in it for a while and come this way together. Practice with pace and flow, and use the close proximity of your mouths and ears to try talking dirty, expressing how good things feel and sharing how turned on you are.

DIFFICULTY ●○○○○ for the giving partner, ●●○○○ for the receiving partner

---

Loving all the body contact but wanting to get more handsy? Have the partner on top gently roll to one side, keeping one leg over the bottom partner to hold them down, and freeing up one arm to really stroke and caress them as they talk dirty in their partner's ear.

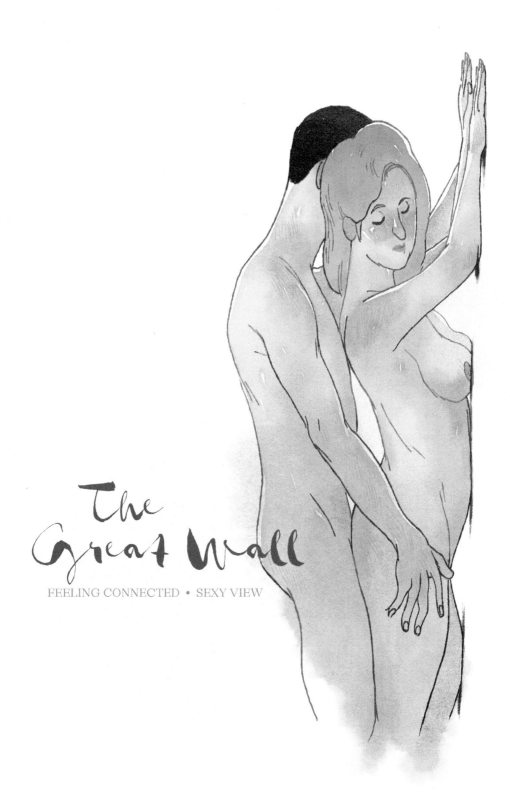

The Great Wall

FEELING CONNECTED • SEXY VIEW

The Great Wall

DESCRIPTION When we think of power, we often think of being thrown up against a wall. This position is a natural progression of that and allows for playing with power and dominance. It can be a great way to feel into your strength, both by capturing your partner and by being caught and resisting. Because you're standing, and so many of your limbs are free, this can feel a bit like upright wrestling. The ultimate result is a lot of body contact and closeness, access to each other's bodies, full-body touch, and plenty of pressing that can feel fantastic.

INSTRUCTIONS You can begin this position in one of two ways: Start out face-to-face and then have the giving partner flip the receiving partner around so they both face in the same direction, or start with the giving partner coming up from behind the receiving partner. If you're experimenting with throw down, have the giving partner firmly push the receiving partner up against the wall, belly to butt, using their full body to hold their partner in place. If you're getting into penetration, it will be from behind, and the wall will provide the resistance to press in. To take it from mild to wild, the giving partner can grab the receiving partner's neck and hair, or wrap their arms around them as they grind and thrust.

WHY YOU'LL LOVE IT This position is all about body contact and energy exchange. Feeling aggressive and strong? Have the giving partner use their body to firmly grab and press against the receiving partner. Feeling softer and more loving? The giving partner can gently move the receiving partner into place, then slowly grind and press against them. This position offers so many options for body exploration and using hot language to get your partner going. Let your hands do the talking or any of the sexy things that come to mind as you are touching your partner. Because this pose is a standing one, you can do it anywhere in your home and even out in public.

DIFFICULTY ●●○○○ for the receiving partner, ●●●○○ for the giving partner

Feeling nervous getting into this position? Let yourself settle into your body, and feel your own physical energy before you connect with your partner. Then, if you are the giving partner, don't be afraid to really push them into the wall. It may feel shocking at first, but that shock can communicate urgency and convey a sense of intention, dominance, and deep desire that will feel good for you both.

The Fold

FONDLING • KISSING

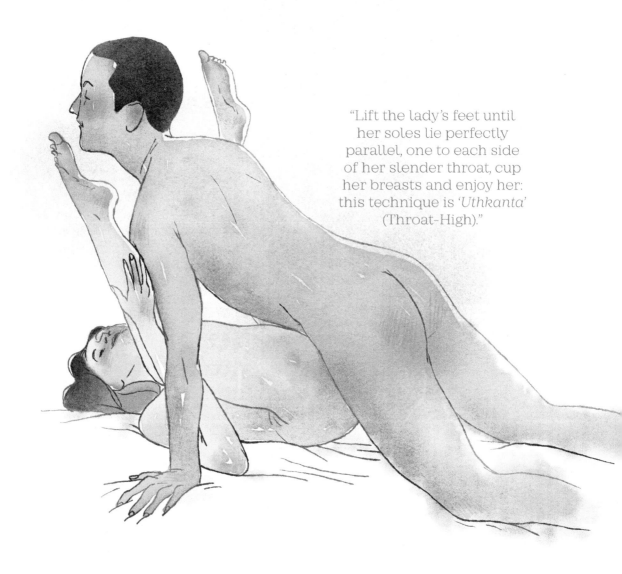

"Lift the lady's feet until her soles lie perfectly parallel, one to each side of her slender throat, cup her breasts and enjoy her: this technique is 'Uthkanta' (Throat-High)."

The Fold

UTHKANTHA (उथ्कन्थ)

DESCRIPTION This position opens the body to new vulnerability for the receiving partner and offers a lot of access to the giving partner. Especially suited for people with flexible hips, the Fold is ideal for exploring dominant energy, as it's a somewhat constraining position and the partner on top can control the pressure, force, and depth of the action. Either partner can be in the receiving position below, so experiment with switching it up according to whoever wants to be forceful in the moment.

INSTRUCTIONS Start in a comfortable spot like a soft bed or squishy couch. Most of the pressure will be on the receiving partner's back, so make sure they have something soft supporting them. The receiving partner lies down on their back and brings their feet up and back by their ears, so their body is folded in half and their tailbone is raised slightly off the ground. The flexibility of their hips will determine the degree of the fold; try it with legs straight and legs bent to find what feels best. The giving partner then connects in penetration with the receiving partner, using the weight of their upper body and hips to grind into them and rock their partner's folded body gently back and forth.

Try this position slowly at first, with the giving partner focusing their energy on holding their partner down, playing with dominant energy and discovering what both partners can enjoy about the pose.

WHY YOU'LL LOVE IT Though it may seem a little intimidating at first or appear physically difficult, this position offers a great physical stretch for many bodies while encouraging intimacy through connection and body weight. It's ideal for playing with energy and power exchange, and in the rock and roll of the flow, it allows for different depths of penetration and can be great for G-spot pleasure.

DIFFICULTY ●●●○○ for the receiving partner, ●●○○○ for the giving partner

Try blindfolding the receiving partner, and begin by caressing their body and placing their legs into position. Excited? Have them prepare by locking their arms around the backs of their thighs so you can enter easily.

V Force

FONDLING • SEXY VIEW

"Grasping the ankles of the round-hipped woman, whose buttocks are like two ripe gourds, raise her beautiful thighs and spread the thigh-joints widely."

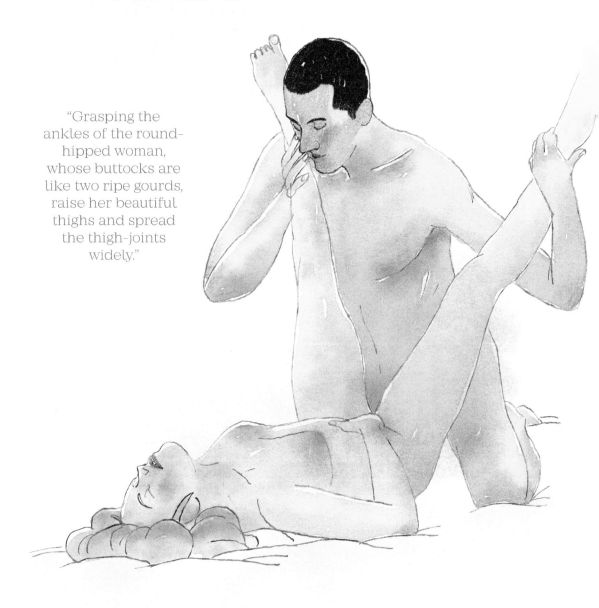

V Force

MADANDHVAJA (मदन्ध्वज)

DESCRIPTION The V Force is another position that works with flexibility in the hips to give play to power, control, and openness. The receiving partner can feel into where this position works for them best, and the giving partner can hold their partner's legs and dominate the moment through moving their limbs around. When we visualize a V position, we think of limbs open and askew, and this pose capitalizes on the heat of that idea and its execution. Feeling splayed and seeing your partner at their most beautiful drives the intensity and sexual excitement of this position.

INSTRUCTIONS This is a position that can be carried out just about anywhere, so it's great when you are looking to get straight to the action. The receiving partner lies on the ground with their legs open at the hips, beginning with feet flat on the floor. The giving partner then moves in on their knees, either upright or with their butt on their heels, depending on their height. Once they have reached the spot where they most want to be, they grab their partner's ankles with their hands and spread their partner's legs up and out on either side of their body in a V shape. The height of the legs will depend on the giving partner's arm strength and the angle that works best for penetration.

WHY YOU'LL LOVE IT This belongs in the family of powerful positions because the sexiness of ankle holding and limb manipulation just can't be denied. As a variation on a more traditional entry position, this one doesn't feel too hard but offers some elements that make it exciting and different from the usual. The weight and intensity is carried by the giving partner, which allows the receiving partner to relax, feel into their body, and enjoy the sensations of having their parts moved for them. For the giving partner, this is a great time to play with power, control, communication, and touch. No need to hold this position for a super-long time, just use your power to take this where you want it to go.

DIFFICULTY ●●○○○ for the receiving partner, ●●○○○ for the giving partner

---

Love holding your partner's ankles or having your body controlled this way? Try flipping this position around! It will also work with the receiving partner on their belly.

The Hijack

FONDLING • TURN-ON

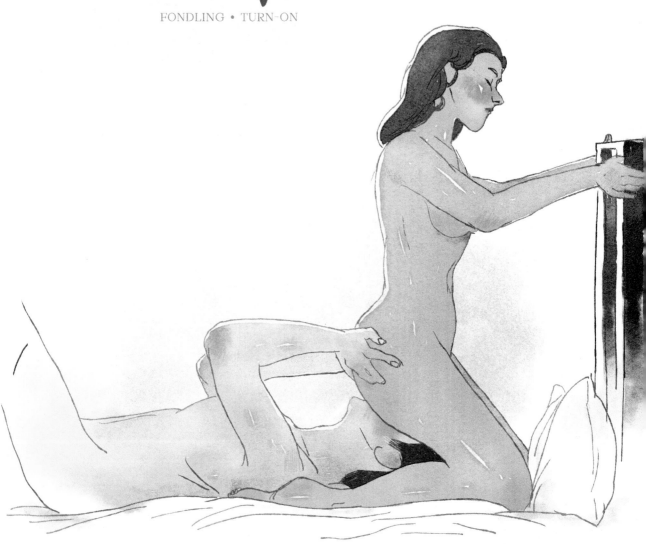

The Hijack

DESCRIPTION The Hijack is the ultimate in powerful oral sex positions and a great option for playing with control, power, dominance, and tease. A relatively simple position to enter, most of the work comes through muscle control and depends on where you are when you attempt it. There are several ways to approach the Hijack, and how you are feeling will characterize the energy you bring to the position.

INSTRUCTIONS This position is best carried out against a wall or near a headboard or sturdy object that the partner on top can hold on to. In this position the partner on top is both giving and receiving, and the vibe you want to achieve will dictate some of the flow. If you are concentrating on your own pleasure, then you are receiving; if you are concentrating on exciting your partner, then you are more on the giving end.

The partner below begins by lying down in a comfortable position, while the partner on top "Hijacks" by straddling their partner's face and playing with the height of their squat until their body is right where they want it. The powerful part of this pose is the control exercised by the partner above as they squat above the partner below; however, the position can easily be brought down onto one's knees on either side of the partner's face below. The top partner can angle their body however they like, using the wall, table, or headboard to hold on and support their weight while they play with the bottom partner and get their O!

WHY YOU'LL LOVE IT There is nothing more powerful than luxuriating in your own pleasure! This position offers the bottom partner a full view of the top partner's gorgeous parts, pushing them to desire and get more turned on. Since the partner on top controls the action, they can fully take control of the pace, flow, movement, and their own enjoyment.

DIFFICULTY ●○○○○ for the partner below, ●●●●○ for the partner above

---

Enjoying the energetic exhibitionism? Have the top partner tilt their body back and give the bottom partner a close-up view as they explore self-touch, enjoying the intimacy of the moment.

Over the Knee

CONTROL • FONDLING

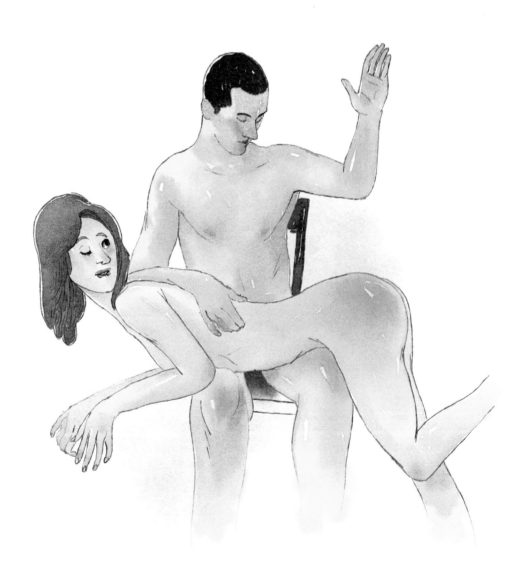

Over the Knee

DESCRIPTION Over the Knee is a classic. And because it's not all about body-to-body penetration, people often forget that it can be a whole lot of fun for foreplay as well as the main event. It's also a great position for playing with power dynamics and all the fun that can come with exhibitionism and hot objectification. Plus, who doesn't love some buns? Don't get caught up in thinking this is just for spanking—the best way to look at this position is as an opportunity for access, power and energy exchange, teasing, and a whole lot of orgasmic possibilities.

INSTRUCTIONS This is one of the simplest positions to enter. The partner providing the lap or knee should start seated in a comfortable spot where their partner can drape across their lower thigh/upper knee area. This can be great to try on a bed where the receiving partner on top can lie flat out or on a chair where they will be fully bent over the lap, hands and feet on the ground.

The receiving partner should take a moment to find a comfortable place-ment for their ribs and belly, so they can breathe and relax and they won't grind into anything particularly painful if they squirm.

WHY YOU'LL LOVE IT This position is sassy and super "cheeky," and it's in the powerful category because it immediately conjures feelings of naughtiness and what we understand as dominant and submissive energy. For the receiving partner, there is much enjoyment to be had in feeling laid out and explored, and for the giving partner, there are all kinds of awesome parts to touch and give you delight. For people with pussies, much can be accessed with hands and fingers in this position, and for folks with cocks, a reach under or down and between can provide a lot of stroking pleasure. You can shift and squirm a lot. See what sexy language comes up for you in this position and let your mind melt into any fantasies that arise.

DIFFICULTY ●○○○○ for the receiving partner, ●●○○○ for the giving partner

---

Find yourself on a chair for this position? The floor will be close, so try rolling the receiving partner onto the floor and moving into the Missionary Push-Up (page 56) or V Force (page 102).

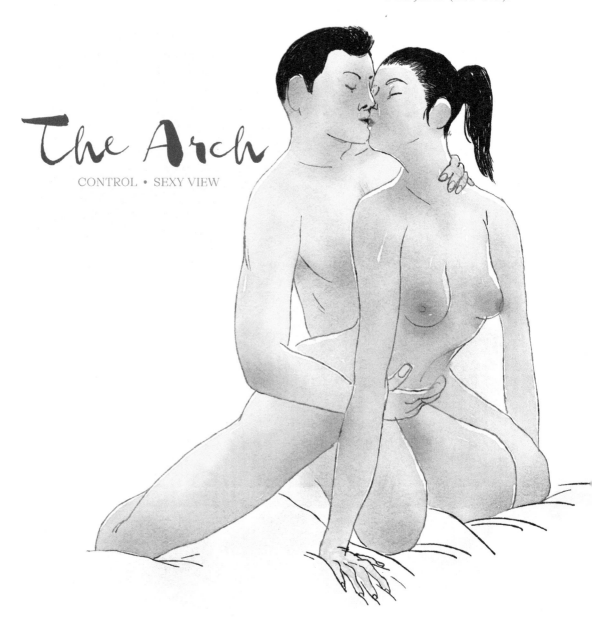

The Arch

CONTROL • SEXY VIEW

"If she lies on her stomach tilting her chin back with your other hand, it is *'Marjara'* (the Cat)."

The Arch

MARJARA (मार्जार)

DESCRIPTION This pose is similar to Classic Doggy (page 120) but uses a slightly different body position to offer options for depth of penetration, closeness, and power play through grabbing, breathing, and gentle force. Because the receiving partner's upper body is more physically supported on their forearms, they are able to achieve a deeper arch in their lower back, making it possible to look back and angle their head so the giving partner can touch and grab their throat, hair, and face.

INSTRUCTIONS The receiving partner begins on a soft surface on their arms and knees, their butt slightly lifted off of their heels. Experimenting with butt height for penetration, the receiving partner may either be up on their hands or down on their forearms. Once you find the connection and flow that feels best for you both, the giving partner reaches up and over their partner's back, grabbing their partner's throat with their flat palm or grabbing a large handful of their partner's hair, deep down at the roots, and giving it a gentle squeeze. The receiving partner will then be tilted back into a gentle lower back arch, their gaze directed either up toward the ceiling or back to one side and at their partner. Experiment with how long you can hold this position and how the level of power and control feels good, evoking a range of sensations from intense to erotic.

WHY YOU'LL LOVE IT This position is energetic and very powerful, combining many elements that folks enjoy: the from-behind doggy position; back, neck, and throat access; and deep penetration. It is especially fun because it allows the receiving partner extra control over the depth and flow of penetration, depending on how much they raise and lower their buns and how tightly they squeeze their thighs together. On the one hand, it can be all about domination and strong power, or on the other hand, it can be about holding, caressing, and deep embodiment. The receiving partner will enjoy being seen and appreciated for their body, and the giving partner will feel that they are getting the best gifts of access, holding, amazing options for touch, and sensational penetration.

DIFFICULTY ●●●○○ for the receiving partner, ●●○○○ for the giving partner

Try closing your eyes in this position, especially when you're moving your bodies closer together through the arch. The receiving partner can experiment with gently tapping on their partner's hand or side when they need a break.

CHAPTER 7

Racy Sex Positions

THE WORD *RACY* TELLS YOU EXACTLY WHAT SOMETHING IN THIS CATEGORY DOES—IT TITILLATES you, making your heart race and your blood pump. Racy stuff is the stuff of fantasy, our deepest turn-ons and curiosities. Bringing an awareness of your fantasies and titillations to your sexual relationship can have a huge impact and up the spice factor instantly.

These sex positions are flattering, exposing, pornographic, and suggestive. Showing off both of your bodies, they provide plenty of hot imagery in the moment as well as visuals to recall and get you aroused later. They push you to notice your own unique brand of sexual performance and give you the chance to experience what is so enticing about watching and being watched by your partner. They also provide opportunities to experience how both you and your partner get turned on by choosing and trying things you think are naughty or risqué.

Try any of these poses when you are feeling the most yourself—for instance, after a date when you've been flirting with one another or whenever you want to push your boundaries and explore fantasies. These are also perfect positions to take out of the bedroom and into the world, as part of the titillation factor might lie in being seen, caught, or feeling taboo.

When you're in the mood for **RACY SEX**, reach out to your partner like this:

1 START WITH SOME SEXY WORDS...

- "I want to fuck you."
- "Please fuck me."
- "I want to get nasty tonight."
- "Tell me your fantasies."
- "Make me feel dirty."
- "I want to feel you inside of me."
- "Let's make our own porno."
- "I like fantasizing about your body and what I want to do to you."

- "You're my little fuck toy."
- "I want to watch you."
- "I can't keep my hands off you."
- "Let's play pretend."
- "I want to spread you open."
- "Give me all of you."
- "Show me everything you want."

2 NEXT, REACH OUT AND TOUCH YOUR PARTNER...

- Start slowly masturbating in front of your partner, enjoying yourself and allowing them to watch and learn.
- Make a little movie of you getting naked or touching yourself, and send it or show it to your partner.
- Be naked and in your favorite position when your partner walks in the door.
- Do a striptease for your partner that ends with you on their lap or leading them to the bed for more fun.
- Fondle your partner slowly and take down their pants, dropping down to enjoy them.
- Reach around behind your partner and run your hands firmly over their most sensitive parts.

- Look for moments to place and move your body seductively: bending over, stretching out, enhancing the parts of you that feel the sexiest.
- Start talking about a fantasy you've always had, holding your partner's gaze while you tell them all the dirty details.
- Take your partner's hand and bring it to your lips. Slowly take one of their fingers and put it in your mouth, sucking softly.
- Leave your partner something sexy you want them to wear or a note describing how you want to see them.

- When you're out in public, find a moment to touch your partner under the table or covertly as you sit side by side. Let your hands wander.

- Do things that bring attention to your mouth: licking your lips, biting your lip, eating slowly, or biting your finger between your teeth.

- Find a moment out in public when you can come up to your partner and gently brush the center of you past their hand(s)—be flirtatious!

3 FINALLY, GET DOWN TO BUSINESS!

THE WATERFALL
(page 114)

THE PORNO PERCH
(page 116)

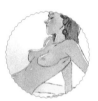

LIE BACK AND RELAX
(page 118)

CLASSIC DOGGY
(page 120)

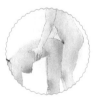

DOWNWARD DOE
(page 122)

EVERYTHING BUTT
(page 124)

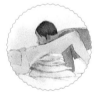

IT'S ALL UP IN THE AIR
(page 126)

THE GET ON DOWN
(page 128)

The Waterfall

RELAXING • SEXY VIEW

The Waterfall

DESCRIPTION This position experiments with deep penetration by turning your bodies on their sides and letting both partners enjoy the sensation of sliding in this way. It gets its name from the way the receiving partner's legs are draped over the giving partner's hips. The Waterfall can be relaxing and casual or high energy and really rough. If you are the giving partner, let your eyes enjoy the beautiful view of your splayed-out partner while you find your flow.

INSTRUCTIONS This is definitely a position you are going to want to try on a big bed or a squishy, comfortable spot with a lot of surface area. The giving partner begins on their side, legs outstretched, either propped up on one arm with their hand supporting their head or with one arm fully outstretched and their head resting on it. The receiving partner then comes in sideways, moving their buns flush to their partner's hips, draping one leg on either side of the giving partner's butt, and sliding into position or letting the giving partner slide into them. In this position, your bodies are perpendicular and the receiving partner's legs are "waterfalling" over the giving partner's body.

WHY YOU'LL LOVE IT The Waterfall is great for penetration, for playing with depth, and grind and finding the G-spot. It may feel like sideways penetration is a little out of the box, and that's the point. Because it's unconventional, it can feel new and exciting and offer you both so many new sensations. One of the hardest kinds of penetration to experiment with can be the very shallow in-and-out, and this position offers great control for playing with that and using varying speed and pace. Your bodies will feel relaxed but still close and connected, and the sexy visuals of your partner grinding into you will charge your arousal and get you both sharing your moans and working each other up before too long.

DIFFICULTY ●○○○○ for the receiving partner, ●●○○○ for the giving partner

Dig this position and its sidesaddle action? Give it a whirl sitting up! You can tilt the entire thing so the partner on their side is lying on their back and the receiving partner is gently sitting in the penetration. With legs outstretched, the receiving partner can grind and ride and enjoy the depth.

The Porno Perch

CARDIO • GRINDING

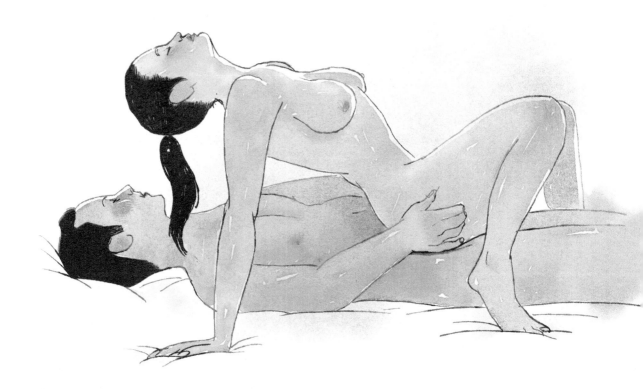

The Porno Perch

DESCRIPTION When my clients talk to me about sexual positions they saw while watching porn, they often describe them as exciting but seemingly beyond reach or maybe even impossible for their bodies. This position is an accessible porn classic that offers a lot in the way of pleasure and can be great fun. Its open and exposing nature gives both partners a chance to feel wild and give in to personal pleasure.

INSTRUCTIONS The giving partner starts out lying flat on their back with their legs outstretched, and the receiving partner then straddles the giving partner's body, facing the giving partner's feet. If you aren't ready for penetration, the receiving partner can lower their body to rest on the giving partner's hips; if you are ready for penetration, the giving partner can raise their arms up and cradle their partner's butt with the palms of their hands. The receiving partner lowers their body onto their partner's hands and leans back, their upper back resting on the giving partner's chest, their head to one side. Once you find your way into the flow, see if it feels best to have the receiving partner lie back or use their hands for support on either side of the giving partner's body.

WHY YOU'LL LOVE IT Oftentimes in positions where the receiving partner is on top, they control much of the flow, pace, and depth of penetration. In this position, however, the receiving partner lies back and gives up control, allowing their weight to be fully supported by the giving partner. This frees up the giving partner to move from the bottom, up, and in and around, enabling them to get rough and wild. This position is a lot of fun and will give both of you the feeling that you're in your own private adult movie. Don't put pressure on yourselves to get this one exactly right, just fully enjoy how much fun it feels to lose yourselves for a bit with one another.

DIFFICULTY ●●●○○ for the receiving partner, ●●○○○ for the giving partner

Feel like this one is wild in a great way? Close your eyes and rock with it, really allowing your body to relax, your breath to deepen, and any wild screams to come out. Notice any moments where you feel nervous or want to hold back and censor yourself? See how you can breathe deeper through and past those barrier moments into your gorgeous body.

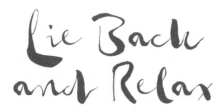

Lie Back and Relax

EYE CONTACT • SEXY VIEW

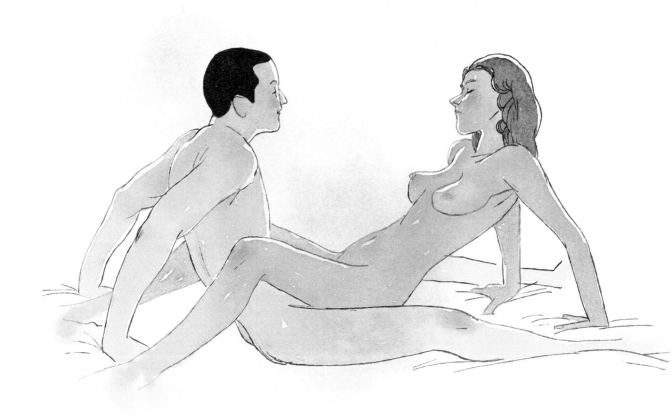

Lie Back and Relax

DESCRIPTION Sometimes the raciest positions are the ones you can really hang out in for a while, getting a great view of one another, grinding, enjoying, and touching yourself at your own pace. This position provides supportive body contact that feels connective but also allows both of you to lie back and settle in, admiring each other's bodies and playing with eye contact. Don't get too caught up in quickening the pace, unless that's exactly what you want. Rather, this position can be perfect for a mellow moment.

INSTRUCTIONS If you're looking to rock and roll in penetration, begin with the penetrating partner in the bottom position, sitting down, legs outstretched in front of them, leaning back on their forearms or against a wall, headboard, or sturdy piece of furniture. The receiving partner then straddles them, legs outstretched as far as they can reach—it's okay if they are bent at the knees or wrapped around the giving partner's low back. The receiving partner then leans back on their arms and both of you enjoy the full view you have as you find your rhythm and thrust.

WHY YOU'LL LOVE IT This position can be just the ticket if you're familiar with the classic cowgirl position but want something more relaxed where you can both stretch out and just connect. Fun for penetration because both of your legs together create a hot mutual squeeze, this also offers a great opportunity for exploring depth. Want deeper penetration? Have the giving partner sit up straighter. Prefer to explore penetration right at the opening? Lay back and then back some more. You'll both love the eye contact and finding ways that you can tease each other. The more casually you settle into your pleasure, the more you'll both feel like you're hanging out in the hottest mellow moment ever.

DIFFICULTY ●●●○○ for the receiving partner, ●○○○○ for the giving partner

---

This position can come as a result of wanting your legs and arms to just stretch and relax, but if you feel too laid out, follow this one into Floating Flower (page 134) or flip it around and reverse it. With so many stimulating possibilities to choose from, you'll have several options for keeping that good flow going.

Classic Doggy

CONTROL • SEXY VIEW

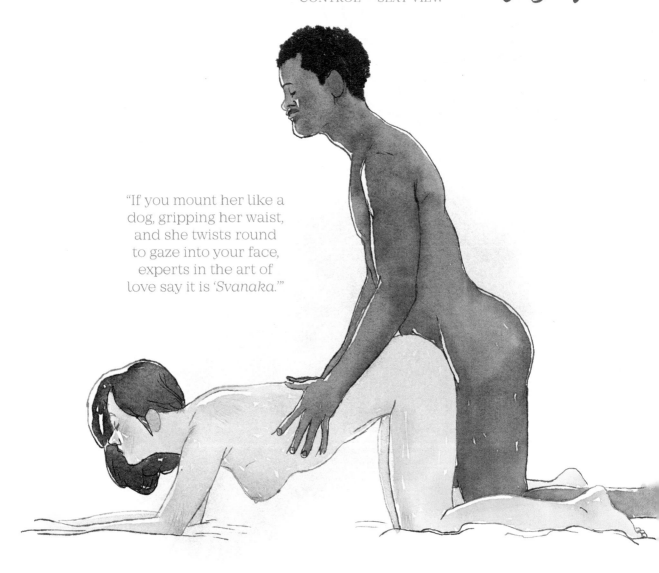

"If you mount her like a dog, gripping her waist, and she twists round to gaze into your face, experts in the art of love say it is *'Svanaka.'*"

Classic Doggy

SVANAKA (स्वनक)

DESCRIPTION There simply cannot be a book on sex positions without including one of the most well-known classics: the Doggy. People love it because it offers a little something for everyone and can be powerful, energetic, intimate, playful, and racy all at once. Explore it more by varying the heights of your bodies: Try starting with the receiving partner on their knees or with their upper body lowered even further.

INSTRUCTIONS A soft surface will be ideal for your knees, though any location can work, and it can be a fun one for spontaneous times. The receiving partner starts out on all fours with their butt in the air. The giving partner slides in behind and, working with comparative pelvis and hip heights, finds their way into grind and penetration. If you are very different heights, experiment with this position off the edge of a bed or a piece of furniture, or try spreading the receiving partner's legs wider so they can get lower. Looking to explore anal sex? To get more control and a better angle, have the giving partner bring one foot up off the floor (keeping the other knee down).

WHY YOU'LL LOVE IT There are many reasons why this position is so popular: the sexy buns view and all the potential butt grabbing; buns serving as a super-hot cushion for penetration; deep penetration with great options for speeding up and slowing down pace and thrust; the incredible view of your partner chest-down on the bed; and the options to grab hair, throats, and shoulders. It has something for everyone and can be a great position for G-spot stimulation, female ejaculation, and self-touch.

DIFFICULTY ●●○○○ for receiving partner, ●●○○○ for giving partner

How do you improve on a classic? Try some impact play or spanking, use this to transition into rough sex, or explore body worship with long, slow caresses over your partner's body. This position can feel like a whole lot of submission, so show your appreciation through touch and enjoyment of their beautiful body.

Downward Doe

CARDIO • ENERGIZING

"If the lady, eager
for love, goes
on all fours,
humping her
back like a doe,
and you enjoy
her from behind,
rutting as though
you'd lost all
human nature,
it is 'Hirana.'"

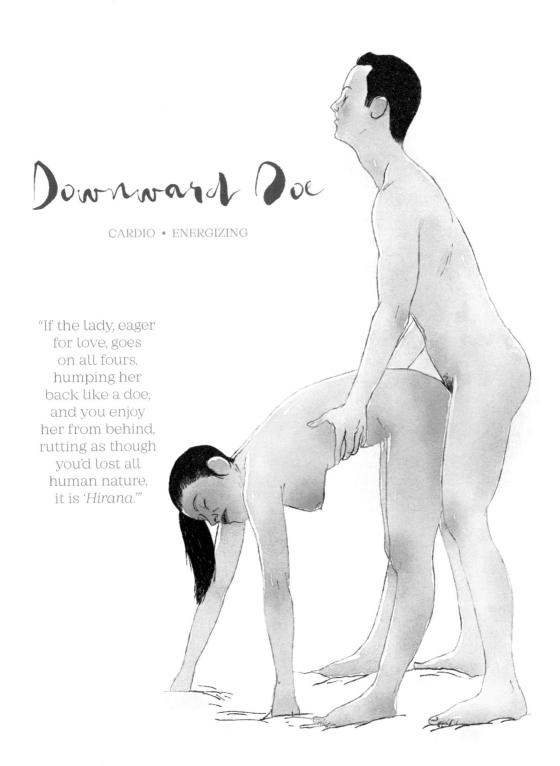

Downward Doe

HIRANA (हरिण)

DESCRIPTION If you love positions that involve penetration from behind and pushing yourself physically during sex, the Downward Doe is for you. It can be challenging to maintain if the receiving partner is not super flexible, but with the giving partner's hands on their hips and butt holding them in the thrust, it can be a lot of fun getting thrown around. Like Doggy in liftoff, this position can be great for spontaneous sex in a variety of places and for nights when you're in the mood for something that showcases a whole lot of body.

INSTRUCTIONS The receiving partner starts out standing and slowly brings their hands to the floor, walking them out just far enough to feel steady supported by the palms of their hands, feet flat on the floor or up on toes if needed. The giving partner moves in from behind, grabbing hold of the receiving partner's hips or butt and using that hold to move into penetration, finding their thrust by rocking back and forth onto the support of the receiving partner's palms. If the receiving partner begins to fall out of the position, try it with them pushing their hands against a wall for greater stability.

WHY YOU'LL LOVE IT This position is definitely a racy one because it can feel a little wild and animalistic for the receiving partner to have their hands on the floor and butt in the air as their partner pushes and thrusts into them. If you're worried that you won't be able to stay in this position for long, don't let that deter you! This position offers a lot in the way of deep penetration, butt fun, grabbing, roughness, and sexual abandon.

DIFFICULTY ●●●●○ for the receiving partner, ●●○○○ for the giving partner

---

Don't forget to breathe! When positions are intense and the thrusting is powerful, our breath can climb up into our throats and get stuck there. If you are the receiving partner, direct your breathing all the way down to your hands and feet. Not only will it help you feel a little more grounded, but it will also help you go deeper into the sensations of the pose.

Everything Butt

GRINDING • RELAXING

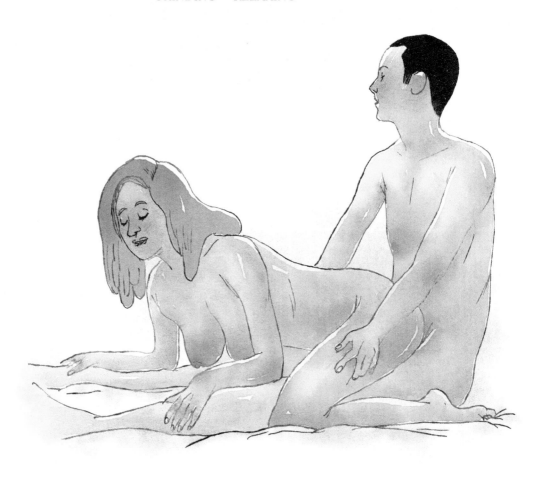

Everything Butt

DESCRIPTION You may be able to tell by now that I love positions that show-case the awesomeness of the butt, and this one is no exception. Super racy in its casual exposure of the length of the receiving partner's body, it's also a position that allows for relaxed closeness and connection. Take it to a high-energy place by ramping up the thrust and grind and turning caressing into grabbing, or follow the slow pace of your energy by really enjoying each other's bodies and taking your time to attain your eventual orgasm.

INSTRUCTIONS The giving partner starts by sitting upright with legs stretched out in front of them and arms by their sides. If you're thinking you'll want to hang out in this one for a while, begin with the giving partner sitting propped up against a wall or headboard—you can always move away from it later. The receiving partner comes in facing away from their partner, as if intending to sit in their lap, with legs on either side of their partner's legs.

As soon as the receiving partner is seated, they then lean forward over their partner's legs, their own legs stretching out behind them alongside the giving partner's waist and back. The receiving partner's upper body will now be fully in the giving partner's lap, and the receiving partner can rest their arms or prop up on their forearms. In this position, the giving partner will need to guide the penetration and the depth and thrust. If the partner on top wants to increase thrust, they can try bending their legs into a frog position behind their partner and using their legs to bring them in and push them out.

WHY YOU'LL LOVE IT Who doesn't love a lap full of buns? There are so many different kinds of fun to be had in this position, from great penetration and exploration with angles to full-body caressing and enjoying all of each other's parts. The receiving partner will love the leg contact and the feel of being in their partner's lap, and the giving partner will love how they can control so much of what feels good for them, while bringing their partner to greater and greater heights of pleasure.

DIFFICULTY ●○○○○ for the receiving partner, ●●●○○ for the giving partner

---

Want to change it up a bit? Try moving away from the wall and having the giving partner lean onto their elbows or all the way back, and see how that impacts the depth and thrust. The giving partner won't be able to caress as much, but this gives the receiving partner a chance to grind a bit more and work their buns.

It's All Up in the Air

ENERGIZING • TURN-ON

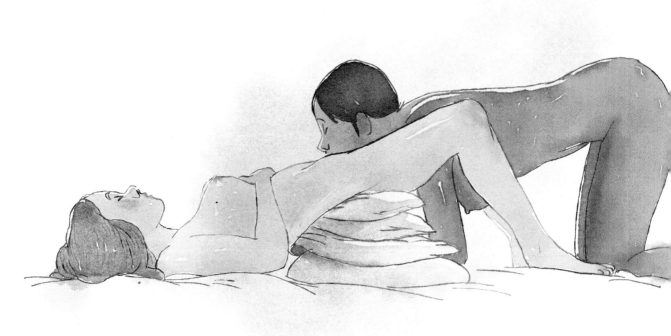

It's All Up in the Air

DESCRIPTION Some of the raciest positions make you the most vulnerable, giving your partner a chance to enjoy you and provide for your pleasure while they explore you at your center. This position allows the receiving partner's body to be relaxed, exposed, and open to pleasure and connection at the same time. It's great for discovering exactly what you want and like and experimenting with communication.

INSTRUCTIONS The receiving partner lies on their back with their knees bent and legs spread out, a pillow positioned lengthwise under their lower back. The giving partner takes in the view and then moves into oral sex. If you're enjoying the feeling of the receiving partner's lifted hips, try experimenting with pillows under the giving partner's chest or hips or giving them something between their legs to grind on and enjoy themselves with.

WHY YOU'LL LOVE IT A common complaint about oral sex is the issue of craned necks and tired hands and tongues. Using pillow support may feel out of the box, but it's an easy way to try different heights and angles for optimum pleasure. Plus, pillows can be malleable and soft props for supporting your body or getting you off. Receiving partners will love how they can relax and worry less about their giving partner's comfort, while giving partners will love how they can move their partner's body exactly where they want it and enjoy being right at their center, surrounded by their pleasure and moans.

DIFFICULTY ●○○○○ for the receiving partner, ●●○○○ for the giving partner

---

Love the height but feel like pillows are unwieldy? Try sex shapes or blankets folded up into broader, firm platforms. Just about anything can be used to prop your body up during sex, as long as it has the firmness or softness you desire.

The Get On Down

CARDIO • SEXY VIEW

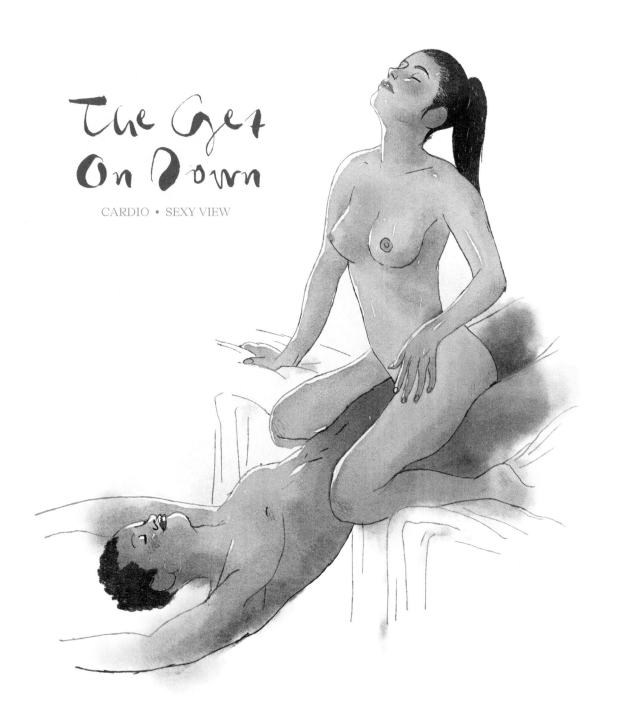

The Get On Down

DESCRIPTION Sometimes you and your partner are in the mood to push your boundaries, challenge yourselves physically, and experience each other in new ways. But even if a position is acrobatic, you still want it to actually feel good. This position will take your bodies to new places together while offering great physical sensation, deep penetration, and a super-fun grind.

INSTRUCTIONS Begin by moving to a bed, couch, or other sturdy piece of furniture. The height you choose for the position will depend on the height of the giving partner, who will be on the floor. The giving partner starts by lying in a bit of a back bend over the edge of the bed (or other piece of furniture); using their hands to support them, they slowly slide down until their shoulders and upper back are resting on the floor. It's important that the giving partner's legs remain relaxed and flat on the bed so they are not balancing all their weight on their neck and back.

The receiving partner, coming from up on the bed or couch, moves in on knees to straddle their partner and then lower onto them in penetration. If the receiving partner feels insecure in the pose, they can move their legs into more of a sitting position. The receiving partner will be responsible for all the depth, grind, and riding in this position, while the giving partner can just lie back and enjoy the feeling and view.

WHY YOU'LL LOVE IT This position is all about the fun and the challenge. You'll get a lot of enjoyment from penetration and body contact, the feeling of wildness and sexual abandon, and the views from both the top and bottom perspectives. Laugh when you want to laugh, feel intensely into your moans, and when you are both ready, collapse in a heap on the floor together. This one is for deeper connection through newness.

DIFFICULTY ●●○○○ for the receiving partner, ●●○○○ for the giving partner

---

Receiving partners, you will notice it's nearly impossible to touch your partner up there. So touch yourself and explore your own gorgeous body. Your partner will love watching you.

CHAPTER 8

Playful Sex Positions

WHEN ASKED TO DESCRIBE THEIR SEXUAL ENERGY, *PLAYFUL* IS ONE OF THE WORDS MY CLIENTS choose most often. It's that bubbling up of fun and silliness, that mischievousness and the sense of creativity and curiosity that emerges and makes you tickle, poke, and tease one another like randy, flirtatious friends. As human beings, we are playful from a very young age, so it's easy to tap into this kind of energy.

These positions are surprising, spontaneous, unexpected, and easygoing, exploring acrobatic possibilities from a place of fun and curiosity. Try them when you're feeling that playful spirit and want to see where that energy can lead you. Playful positions allow you to concentrate on your own pleasure and are less focused on deep connection with your partner, so they can be great for quickies and those moments when you have less time to devote to full sexual lovemaking. They are also ideal for trying spontaneity and having sex in all sorts of locations beyond the bedroom.

When you're in the mood for **PLAYFUL SEX**, reach out to your partner like this:

1 START WITH SOME SEXY WORDS...

- "Let's play."
- "I like you."
- "Let's get silly."
- "Wanna fool around?"
- "Let's wrestle."
- "You make me feel giddy inside."
- "Let's have some fun."

- "You're my best friend."
- "I'm in a playful mood."
- "I've been thinking about you all day."
- "I'm so excited about you."
- "There's something I want to try."
- "Let's play a game . . ."

2 NEXT, REACH OUT AND TOUCH YOUR PARTNER...

- Use a nickname for your partner in playful way.
- Describe your playful energy to your partner—tell them how good it feels and where you feel it. Grab your partner around the waist or hips, and let your hands rest there.
- Gently tickle your partner in neutral places like the lower back, the knees, or the back of the neck.
- Pull your partner close to you with a smile.
- Grab your partner's buns.
- Kiss your partner on the nose.
- Slow dance without any music, just rocking together in silence.
- Begin to wrestle playfully with your partner.

- Start a gentle pillow fight around your partner's chest and shoulders.
- Grab both sides of your partner's face for a big-lipped smooch.
- Come up behind your partner and whisper in their ear.
- Trace the outline of your partner's face with your fingers.
- Let your hands run along your partner's body and give them gentle squeezes all over.
- Throw your arms around your partner and lift them slightly in the air.
- Come up behind your partner and give them little thrusting humps—let yourself enjoy it!
- Roll around with each other, and take turns flipping each other over.

3 FINALLY, GET DOWN TO BUSINESS!

THE FLOATING FLOWER
(page 134)

THE ROOTED FLOWER
(page 136)

STAND AND DELIVER
(page 138)

THE GET A GRIP
(page 140)

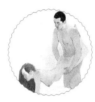

GET IN WHERE YOU FIT IN
(page 142)

THE LOCK BOX
(page 144)

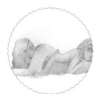

THE ULTIMATE TEASE
(page 146)

TAKE A LAP
(page 148)

THE SAFETY SCISSORS
(page 150)

The Floating Flower

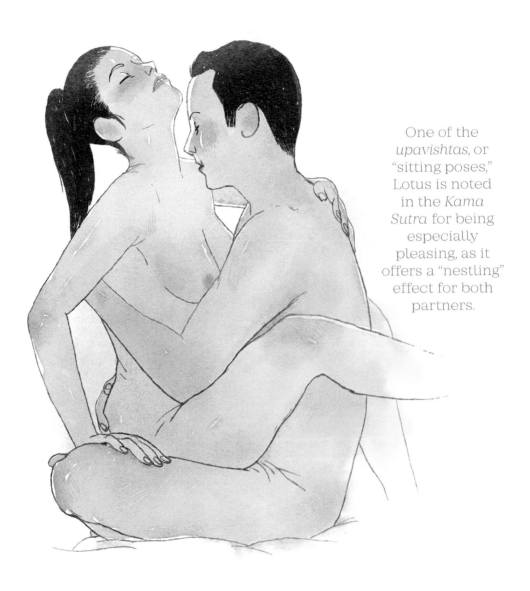

One of the *upavishtas,* or "sitting poses," Lotus is noted in the *Kama Sutra* for being especially pleasing, as it offers a "nestling" effect for both partners.

The Floating Flower

LOTUS (बसिनी)

DESCRIPTION The Floating Flower is a classic of the *Kama Sutra*. It's unique in the way your bodies will grind, rock, and rub, while still leaving ample space to look at and touch one another.

INSTRUCTIONS The giving partner sits crossed-legged and then the receiving partner climbs into their partner's lap, wrapping legs around their partner's waist so pelvises touch and penetration is at its deepest. While this position will feel less like thrusting and more like a back-and-forth, rocking-and-rolling groove, the depth makes it a very worthwhile position for both involved.

Start slowly and allow for that playful, exploratory energy to get your momentum going. "How do our bodies fit?" "How can I tease you by moving closer and playing with eye contact, then moving away and closing my eyes to enjoy my pleasure and the view?"

You may like to try this position on a soft surface that allows you to sink into it and be supported as you grind, but doing it on a hard or firm surface will give you more motion. Either way, make sure something soft or smooth is beneath the bottom partner, as uncomfortable friction and/or burn can definitely occur!

WHY YOU'LL LOVE IT The Floating Flower is a classic for a reason. It's fun, connective, and leaves your hands free for touching, grabbing, and stroking. It's great when you want to look at each or move ear-to-ear for sexy talk, heavy breathing, and those giggles that can be part of your playful self.

People with clitorises will love it because the upright position allows for both deep penetration and clitoral stimulation. Also, the partner on top holds most of the control, so if you feel like teasing and showing off or playing with the energy between you, it's all in your hands (or pelvis).

The penetrating partner will love having a lap full of buns, a great view of the receiving partner, and lots of pleasurable grinding and rubbing. Enjoy the depth of penetration and see if you can to lean back and grind deeper, or simply cradle your partner and drink in the moment.

DIFFICULTY ●●○○○ for the seated partner, ●●●○○ for the partner on top

---

Up the intensity by having the bottom partner open their legs wider to create more space for you to be pelvis-to-pelvis. Also, try having the top partner raise one leg, bracing on the floor or bed behind them. This allows for openness in the hips and more connection, not to mention a great view of all the parts at play.

The Rooted Flower

KISSING • TEASING

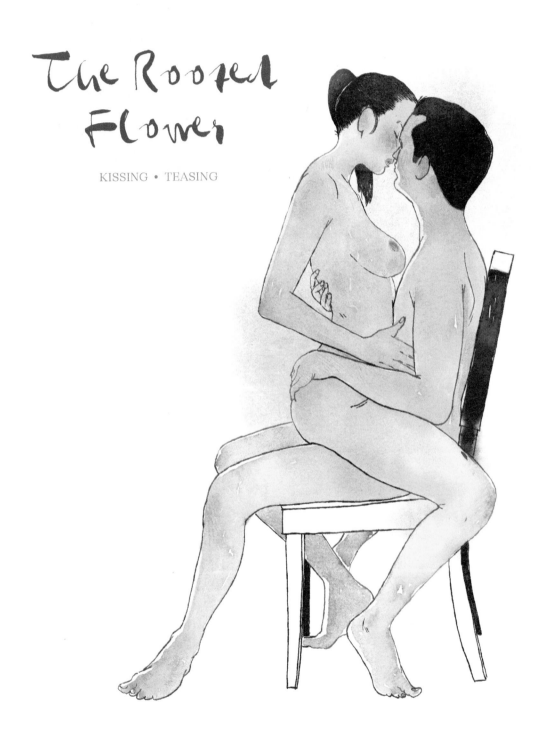

The Rooted Flower

VARIATION ON LOTUS (उपकरक पद्मिनी)

DESCRIPTION While the Floating Flower (page 134) is a classic *Kama Sutra* position, it can be difficult for bodies with tight hips. The Rooted Flower is raised up off the floor with legs dangling instead of being crossed around one another.

INSTRUCTIONS Find a sturdy chair without arms, an ottoman, or a small table; having a back to the chair or a wall behind you can be helpful as well. The bottom partner begins by sitting in the chair with both feet on the floor. The top or receiving partner straddles the bottom partner's lap and allows their legs to dangle. If the top partner can touch the floor with their toes, they can push off, lower down, and possibly get a good bounce.

The partner on top controls much of the depth, stroke, and pace, but the partner below can get feisty, grabbing and pulling closer, thrusting upward, and generally enjoying the feeling of the grind and being ridden.

WHY YOU'LL LOVE IT This position offers a lot of appealing options, from the approach to the different kinds of movement while you're in it. The receiving partner can have fun with the approach, doing a little sexy dance, crawling toward the giving partner while making eye contact, and then teasing as they straddle their partner's lap. If you are using a chair with a back, the receiving partner can hold on and really feel like they are riding the giving partner. The seated partner can grab handfuls of buns, get face level with breasts, and support their partner's body as they rock back and forth and lean back to play with the depth of penetration.

Much like Floating Flower, this position offers chances for deep penetrative strokes, clitoral stimulation, reach-around grabbing, touching of chests and licking of nipples, and breathing in each other's ears, on collarbones, and on necks. You can also determine when you want eye contact and connection and when you want to cuddle in, drop deeper into your body, and just rock and roll.

DIFFICULTY ●●●○○ for the partner on top, ●●○○○ for the seated partner below

---

If you're in a chair with a back or solid support for the bottom partner, the top partner can try rocking their body back, lifting their legs, and resting them on the giving partner's shoulders. Have the giving partner support the receiving partner's lower back while they push their butt deeper into the giver's lap. In this leaned-back position, the receiving partner will have a little more room to explore self-touch in ways that feel awesome. And, of course, the giving partner will love the view.

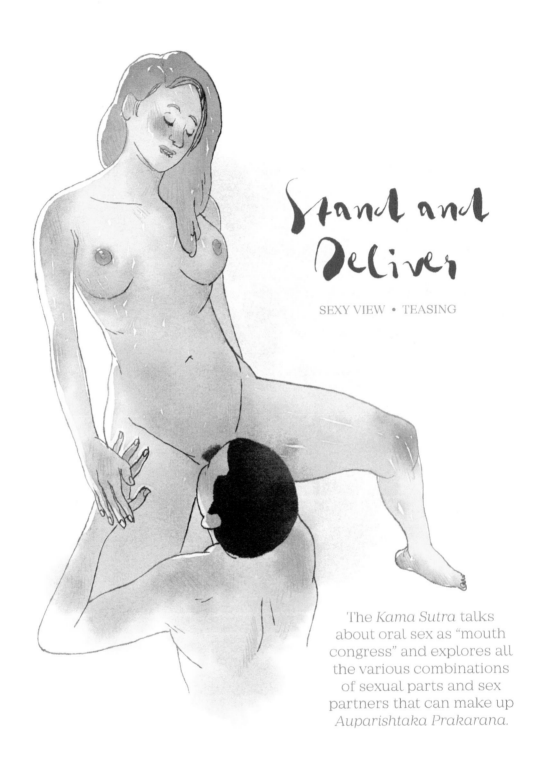

Stand and Deliver

SEXY VIEW • TEASING

The *Kama Sutra* talks about oral sex as "mouth congress" and explores all the various combinations of sexual parts and sex partners that can make up *Auparishtaka Prakarana*.

Stand and Deliver

DESCRIPTION This position is incredibly powerful for both the giver and receiver in unique ways. Through offering your body to be consumed by your partner's mouth, you hold so much allure and are physically presenting what you want and choosing when and how you get it.

INSTRUCTIONS The receiving partner stands and places one raised leg on a bed, couch, ottoman, or low table (feel free to get creative with the location), and the giving partner moves close to and underneath the standing partner's waiting body. Legs tucked comfortably beneath them or sitting crossed-legged, the giving partner takes their partner into their mouth.

WHY YOU'LL LOVE IT Oftentimes people think of standing oral sex positions as disempowering, but they can be so much fun and so powerful for both parties. In this epitome of a playful posture, the standing partner can playfully tease and show off their beautiful body as they sensually encourage their partner to connect to it with their mouth. The giving partner can also tease with how close they get, showing what they want to do with their tongue and even their fingers. Once connected in the posture, both partners have their hands free for stroking their own bodies or touching all over one another. It's a great position for when you're feeling frisky and want to play with control.

Notice how it feels to show your body to your partner. Connect to your breathing, and feel how your heartbeat quickens. How does it feel to have them look at you, imagining what they might do with you? What do you love about your body, and how can you playfully show that off? Maybe you want to close your eyes and feel the energy coursing through you. For the giving partner, this can be a posture of great body worship; how can you show through eye contact, touch, and with your mouth how much you want your partner? Let yourself be cheeky and teasing, and feel the energy of your arousal grow within.

DIFFICULTY ●●●○○ for the standing partner, ●○○○○ for the kneeling partner

Is it all feeling so good that you get weak in the knees? Try grabbing for a chair or the edge of the couch to let your body relax into it. Use your remaining free hand to run over your body, and notice how your skin feels and how your body is getting warmer. Let your hand come to rest in your partner's hair or playfully touch their ears or neck with encouragement and desire.

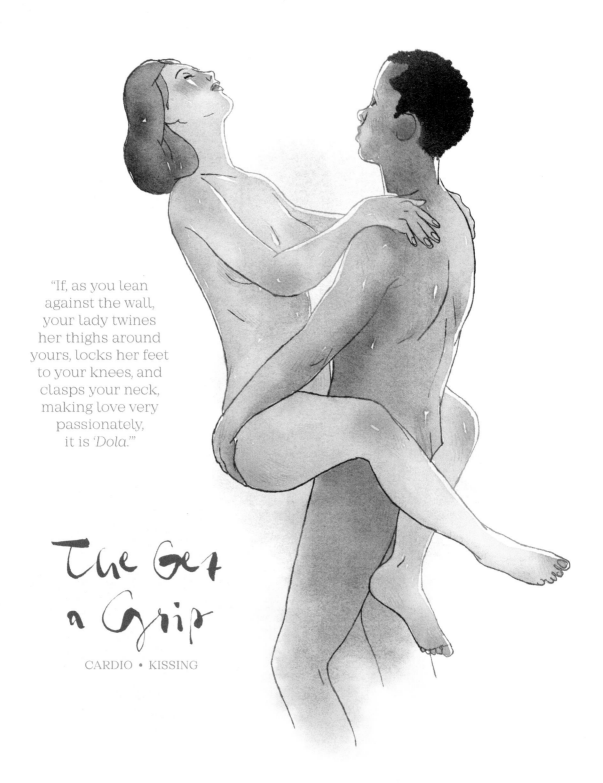

"If, as you lean against the wall, your lady twines her thighs around yours, locks her feet to your knees, and clasps your neck, making love very passionately, it is *'Dola.'*"

The Get a Grip

CARDIO • KISSING

The Get a Grip

DOLA, OR "SWING" (दोला)

DESCRIPTION This position is for when your desire is too strong and you just can't make it to the bed, or you're simply in the mood for adventure and want to share your passion standing up.

INSTRUCTIONS The standing partner begins with their back to a wall or against the back of a couch or chair. The hanging partner starts with wrapping their arms around their partner's neck to support their lower body, then they wrap one leg around their partner's waist, bringing the other leg up to lock with the first leg at the ankles. When the hanging partner feels set in the position, they can let go and lean back, supported by their partner's arms.

If you're getting into penetration, move into the position first, and then find a good angle for entry. The standing partner grips under the buns of the hanging partner and uses their arm strength to help with grinding and bouncing their partner up and down. Meanwhile, the hanging partner uses their thigh strength to find movement that feels good for them.

WHY YOU'LL LOVE IT The Get a Grip is a super-fun position to try when you are both feeling randy and experimental. It engages the whole body and works different muscles than the usual ones. While this position isn't the most relaxed, it gives both partners a chance to feel strong and powerful and silly and playful at the same time.

For the giving partner, it can feel great to experience the different angles you can achieve in penetration and to have your hands full of buns as you support and move your partner on your body. For the receiving partner, enjoy the hang! Notice how much fun it can be to swing from your partner and grip them with your powerful thighs. You can use the squeeze of your thighs and vary your arm positioning to get higher or lower on your partner, depending on how deep you want the penetration to be and what kind of grinding and other movements feel best.

DIFFICULTY ●●●●● for the hanging partner, ●●●○○ for the standing partner

Finding Get a Grip fun but too hard to maintain for very long? Turn around and see if it's easier when the receiving partner can press their toes and feet into the wall, or prop them up on the edge of the couch. If you're laughing and giggling, go with it! This position is exciting, funny, and wild! Throw back your head and let that animated, silly energy come out—that's your playful nature!

Get In Where You Fit In

CARDIO • SEXY VIEW

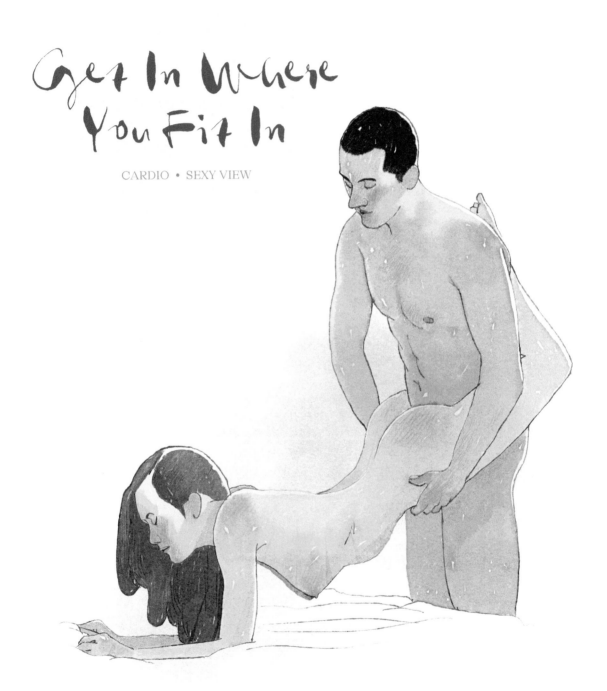

Get In Where You Fit In

DESCRIPTION This position allows for varying levels of penetration or grinding and offers access that can be difficult to achieve with both partners lying down. It's also a huge visual treat for the standing partner, and it gives them a chance to control the speed and pace, as well as tease their partner by playfully moving their body and their partner's body in the pose.

INSTRUCTIONS The receiving partner begins by lying on their belly across a small ottoman, stable chair, or the width of a bed with their legs extended in a V. If they have good upper body support, they can let their arms dangle or rest on the ground. If extra support is necessary, they can use their arms to hold their upper body parallel with their legs. Ideally, the receiving partner should be lying at approximately the same height as the giving partner's waist. The giving partner then moves in between the receiving partner's legs, holding the receiving partner above the knees. From here, the receiving partner's legs can be spread out more or tightened, depending on what feels best for both partners.

WHY YOU'LL LOVE IT This position is all about getting close. If you love Doggy (page 120), then you will enjoy how this position gives a lot of possibility for going deep while still allowing for control. The standing partner is in between legs the whole time, even when they're not penetrating, and that can allow for a lot of fun teasing, leg touching, and body wriggling from the partner lying down.

It may seem like you need to have a lot of flexibility to feel great in this position, but that isn't the case: The varying ways your bodies will fit together truly allows the standing partner to really get in there, which can be incredibly playful, both in assuming the position and in moving, grinding, and penetration once you're in deep.

This position offers the ultimate sexy view, which allows for butt wiggling, teasing, and the playful seduction of the rear end. No doubt the standing partner will love how much control and access this gives them.

DIFFICULTY ●●●●○ for the standing partner, ●●○○○ for the partner lying down

---

Depending on height and how you use props and furniture to help your bodies align, the Get In Where You Fit In can be a great position for anal sex as well as vaginal sex and grinding. Is the receiving partner having a tough time keeping their legs open in a wide V? Try having them bend their knees, and see if that allows their hips to open further in ways that feel good.

The Lock Box

FONDLING • TURN-ON

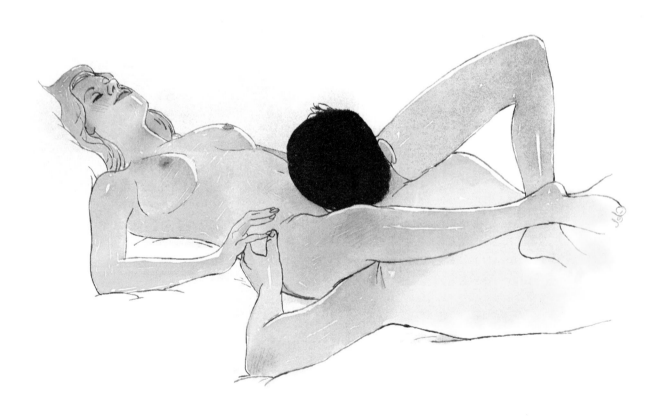

The Lock Box

AMRACHUSHITA (अमरचुषितं)

DESCRIPTION Designed for partners with pussies to be on the receiving end, this pose is referred to in the *Kama Sutra* as *Amrachushita*, or "Sucking the Mango." This position can be fun for folks of all bodies, as the receiving partner gets to control and tease by locking their legs around their partner's head and upper shoulders.

INSTRUCTIONS This is a relaxed position that can follow kissing, fondling, and working your way down your partner's body. The giving partner places their head comfortably between their partner's legs, leaning to one side, arms reaching toward their partner's lower body and butt, head resting on their partner's inner thigh. The receiving partner then clasps their legs behind their partner's back, resting their clasped feet just below the head.

WHY YOU'LL LOVE IT This position is really playful because it allows the receiving partner to bring the giving partner's head closer to their body or move it further away to tease and control the pace and intensity of oral sex. Receiving partner: Want to keep your partner mere inches from your pussy to experience the intensity of your turn-on? Bring your inner thighs closely together to push their head out and hold them in place. Orgasm is also super erotic in this position, as the giving partner gets to feel thighs shake, butt muscles shiver, and legs clasp tighter as pleasure shifts.

This position is really designed for the receiving partner but offers hot visuals for the giving partner and a chance for them to be super close to their partner's beautiful body. Notice how both partners get chances to tease in this position, and feel how the position offers moments of connection in between.

DIFFICULTY ●○○○○ for both partners

Notice how this position mimics wrestling and can seem like having your partner in a modified headlock? Allow yourself to drop deeply into feelings of power and playfulness, and use those feelings to help you choose your own pleasure in this pose. If you are the giving partner, use your hand when it feels fun to try. In addition, notice where your partner is leading you. Are they allowing you to take small "sips" of pleasure, urging you to enjoy more of them, or are they really wanting you to work for it? Follow that energy.

The Ultimate Tease

FONDLING • TEASING

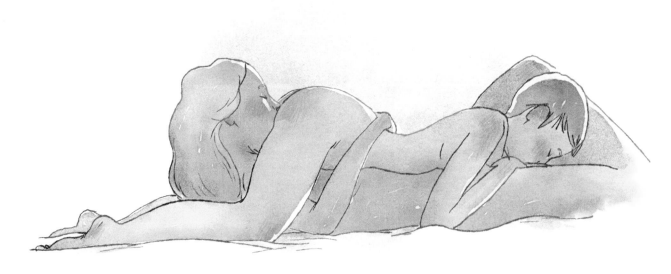

The Ultimate Tease

VARIATION ON THE CLASSIC 69

DESCRIPTION The 69 allows both partners to go down on each other at the same time. Clients frequently describe it as "distracting, overwhelming, and confusing" and often ask me how to enjoy it more, because it seems like it should be so much fun! This slight spin on the position allows for a more playful energy where each person focuses on their own pleasure and takes what they most want from the pose and the experience.

INSTRUCTIONS Decide who will go above and below and find a comfortable and relatively soft place to lie down. Firm surfaces like a floor can be suitable, but keep in mind that you might be in this position for a while, and all the squirming and rubbing could easily result in rug burn and sore elbows and knees. I invite each of you to experiment with both top and bottom position.

To start, the bottom partner lies on their back and the top partner straddles them on all fours, their head facing their partner's feet. Now the playful twist: Do not immediately lower your mouth or body down to your partner. Play with them. See how you can hover over your partner's parts, breathing, teasing, and keeping your parts a bit distant from their face.

WHY YOU'LL LOVE IT In the Ultimate Tease, you are focusing completely on your own pleasure. What are you enjoying more: your partner's mouth on you or using your mouth to tease them? Choose which you prefer, and really immerse yourself in all the sensations of that act.

If you are on bottom, use your arms and play with distance and control by holding your partner right where you want them, grabbing and enjoying the feel of their body.

Try closing your eyes and bringing your breath down to the part of your body where you're feeling the strongest sensation. Notice how your breath intensifies what you feel and how closing your eyes helps your mind drop into your body.

DIFFICULTY ●●○○○ for both partners

Still struggling with focus and having a hard time teasing your partner because they want to get right at you? Tie the bottom partner down to the bed or chair, and control the action from up top. Bring your parts over their face for a great view, and drop them to your partner's mouth when you want stimulation, but this time focus mainly on your partner, feeling their want for you and noticing how that turns you on and brings out your playful energy.

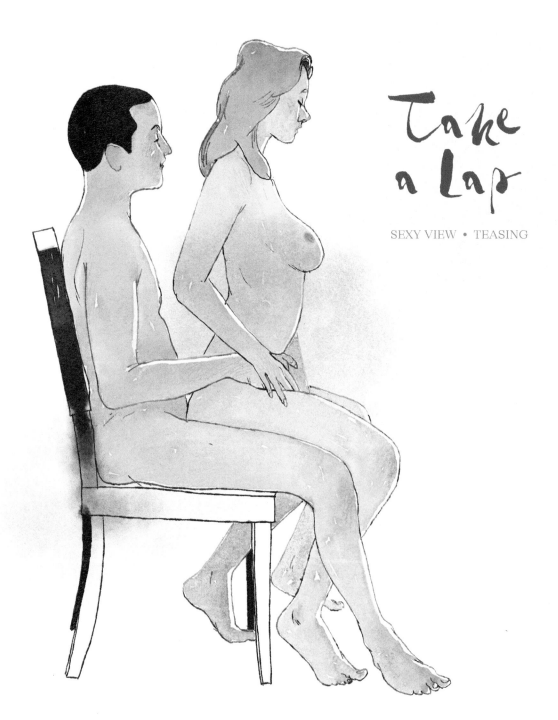

Take a Lap

SEXY VIEW • TEASING

Take a Lap

DESCRIPTION Who doesn't love a lap dance? This position utilizes seductive movement and the appeal of a lap full of buns to charge the energy and give you both a super-fun grind.

INSTRUCTIONS The bottom partner sits on a nice wide couch or bed or on a stable chair with their feet on the floor. The top partner backs their buns onto the bottom partner's lap. The bottom partner can experiment by closing their legs or spreading them open in a small V shape, and the top partner can keep their legs together, tilting slightly forward, or bring their legs to either side of their partner's waist and tucking them back into a crouch. Explore what feels best and is most comfortable for you and your partner's bodies.

WHY YOU'LL LOVE IT One of the best parts of this position is just getting into it. Whether you crawl across the floor to your waiting partner or dance for them, running your hands over your body, there are countless options for what I like to call "the approach." A good portion of the playful energy here lies in how the top partner brings their buns to rest in their partner's lap and how the bottom partner beckons them to do it, showing their desire.

If you're playing with penetration, each of these variations lets you control how deep you go, the pace, and the grind. For tighter and shallower penetration, have the receiving partner keep their legs together while the penetrating partner spreads into the V. To get deeper and allow for more action, do the reverse: The penetrating partner's legs stay together, and the receiving partner's legs spread open.

The chance to watch and be watched can be extremely exciting. If having your partner's eyes on you feels too intense, face away from them and try slowly running your hands over your beautiful body. When you face them, allow yourself to keep your eyes closed, dropping into your body's playful energy. Feel into the sexiness of your teasing, and notice how that energy grows as you move closer to your partner.

DIFFICULTY ●○○○○ for the seated partner, ●●●○○ for the partner on top

---

Experiment by having the bottom partner lean back and the top partner lean forward. When the top partner leans forward, they give their partner an even better view of their butt while they explore different depths and brace themselves to allow for more movement.

The Safety Scissors

ENERGIZING • SEXY VIEW

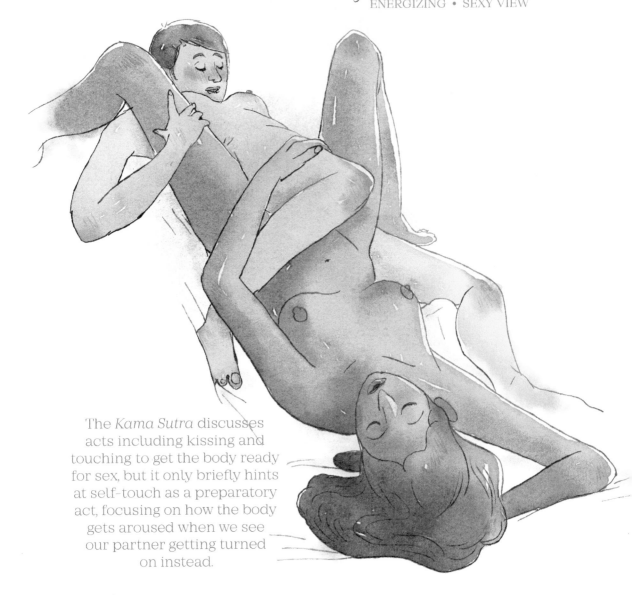

The *Kama Sutra* discusses acts including kissing and touching to get the body ready for sex, but it only briefly hints at self-touch as a preparatory act, focusing on how the body gets aroused when we see our partner getting turned on instead.

The Safety Scissors

DESCRIPTION One of the best ways to learn what your partner wants is by watching them touch their own body and seeing how they get turned on. Often we think of masturbation as a solo experience, but this position introduces all the possibilities of touching yourself as a partnered activity. Watching your partner become aroused can be incredibly arousing for you as well, but it is equally arousing to be watched.

INSTRUCTIONS Both partners lie on their backs on a comfortable, soft surface—a bed or couch works best. You begin lying next to one another, heads in opposite directions. The person with the shorter legs then drapes one leg over their partner's chest and to one side of their head. The partner with the longer legs then drapes their same leg over their partner's chest as well. In this position, you will look like two overlapping and intertwined V shapes. Depending on the lengths of your legs, both bodies will turn gently toward each other, moving slightly onto their sides. Angle yourself toward your partner so you get a great view of their hot body as they pleasure themself.

WHY YOU'LL LOVE IT What is more exciting and playful than watching your partner get turned on? This position allows for all the fun of mutual masturbation with a twist that helps you stay connected to each other's bodies and energies. Experiment with placing a pillow beneath your head so you are propped up, looking your partner in the eye, or see how you feel lying back for less eye contact, therefore feeling more on your own, though at the same time together.

Touching yourself while your partner watches is a moment ripe with tease and titillation. Watch what they do when you move and touch yourself in certain ways. Listen to their breath quicken and feel the muscles of their legs contract and stretch as they get increasingly aroused. This position is the ultimate learning playground for each partner. Notice how your partner touches themself, and take mental notes of things you observe and want to try on them in the future.

DIFFICULTY ●○○○○ for both partners

Close your eyes, and feel into how you like to touch yourself. There is no right or wrong way to enjoy your body, and the more you let yourself go, the more your partner gets to observe and learn from your pleasure. If you feel yourself moving toward their body and wanting more connection, allow yourself to roll onto your side, grip their leg between your thighs for a slow, luxurious grind, and just lose yourself in whatever sensations feel amazing.

TAKE A CHANCE Roll a six-sided die. Then roll it again. Whatever comes up, give it a try.

	POSITION	MOOD	PAGE
⚀⚀	THE ARCH	POWERFUL	108
⚀⚁	CLASSIC DOGGY	RACY	120
⚀⚂	DOWNWARD DOE	RACY	122
⚀⚃	EVERYTHING BUTT	RACY	124
⚀⚄	THE FLOATING FLOWER	PLAYFUL	134
⚀⚅	THE FOLD	POWERFUL	100
⚁⚀	THE FULL FRONTAL	ENERGETIC	86
⚁⚁	THE FULL PRESS	POWERFUL	96
⚁⚂	THE G HUNTER	POWERFUL	94
⚁⚃	THE GET A GRIP	PLAYFUL	140
⚁⚄	GET IN WHERE YOU FIT IN	PLAYFUL	142
⚁⚅	THE GET ON DOWN	RACY	128
⚂⚀	THE GREAT WALL	POWERFUL	98
⚂⚁	THE HIJACK	POWERFUL	104
⚂⚂	THE IN-BETWEEN	INTIMATE	58
⚂⚃	IT'S ALL UP IN THE AIR	RACY	126
⚂⚄	THE KNEELING MISSIONARY	INTIMATE	62
⚂⚅	THE LEG UP	ENERGETIC	82
⚃⚀	LIE BACK AND RELAX	RACY	118
⚃⚁	THE LOCK BOX	PLAYFUL	144

Index

CPSIA information can be obtained
at www.ICGtesting.com
Printed in the USA
BVOW07s1112271016
R7556500001B/R75565PG465627BVX1B/1/P